Immune
Recovery

The Pathway to Building Healthy Immunity

Dr. Anna Mike Marla

Table of Contents

IMMUNE SYSTEM RECOVERY I

FREE BONUS 10

PREFACE 11

INTRODUCTION 15

CHAPTER 1 20

    THE HUMAN IMMUNE SYSTEM 20

    FUNCTION OF THE IMMUNE SYSTEM 20

        How the Immune System Functions 21

    HUMAN IMMUNE SYSTEM MAKE UP 25

        The Bone Marrow 26

        The Thymus 28

        Lymphocytes 29

        Lymph Nodes and Spleen 32

    WAYS TO KEEP THE IMMUNE SYSTEM HEALTHY 36

        Eat a Healthy Diet Plan 37

        Get a lot of Quality Sleep 40

        With regards to Alcohol, Practice Moderation 41

        Keep Stress in Check 42

        Keep Symptoms of Chronic Conditions in Order 44

        Don't Smoke Cigars 45

        Exercise Regularly (Outdoors, When Possible) 46

    PREPARE TO STRENGTHEN YOUR IMMUNE SYSTEM 49

        Your Social Life can Make You Stronger 49

        Regular Sex is Helpful 51

        Processed Foods Diet deprive the Body of Nutrients 51

        Optimize Your Diet for Optimal Immune Function 52

        Fight Disease with Laughter 53

        Multivitamin Can Help 53

        Pets are a Boon to Immunity 54

        Stress 54

Be Positive to Improve Immune Response 55

CHAPTER 2 57

NATURAL WAYS TO BOOST THE IMMUNE SYSTEM 57

Lessen Your Stress Levels... 58
Reduce your Alcohol Intake. 58
Ensure You Get Your A-B-C-D-Es... 59
Try Colostrum 59
Eat lots of Vegetables... 60
Herbs & Supplements 60
Exercise regularly 61
Get adequate sleep 61
Start to eat Mushrooms 61
Quit smoking 62
Step into the sun! 62
Stay Active... 64
Watch your daily diet 65
Stick to the top of the stress 66
Get enough sleep.. 68

BE STRATEGIC ABOUT SUPPLEMENTS.. 69

CHAPTER 3 70

FOODS THAT BOOST AND INCREASE YOUR IMMUNE SYSTEM 70

Elderberry 70
Mushrooms.. 72
Acai Berry 73
Oysters 74
Watermelon 75
Watermelon Nutrition... 76
Wheat Germ 77
Yogurt.. 78
Spinach.. 79
Tea... 80
Sweet Potatoes 81

Broccoli 83

Garlic 84

Miso soup 86

Chicken Soup 87

Pomegranate 89

Ginger 90

OTHER FOODS THAT BOOST AND INCREASE YOUR IMMUNE SYSTEM 92

Elderberry 92

Mushrooms 95

Acai Berry 96

Oysters 97

Watermelon 98

Wheat Germ 99

Yogurt 101

Spinach 102

Tea 103

Sweet Potatoes 104

Broccoli 106

Garlic 107

Miso soup 108

Chicken soup 109

Pomegranate 111

Ginger 112

CHAPTER 4 .... **115**

IMMUNE BOOSTING FOODS, TONICS & TEAS. 115

FRUITS 116

Coconuts & Coconut Oil 116

Berries 117

Citrus Fruits 118

Apples 118

TEAS 119

Ginger Tea 119

Holy Basil (Tulsi Tea) 120

    Mint *120*

    Chamomile *120*

    Lavender *121*

VEGETABLES 122

    Cabbage *123*

    Garlic *123*

    Red Pepper *124*

    Spinach *124*

TINCTURES & EXTRACTS 125

    Astragalus *126*

    Oregano Oil *127*

    Mushroom Extracts *127*

    Echinacea extract *128*

HERBS 128

    Oregano *129*

    Turmeric *129*

    Ginger *130*

    Licorice Root *130*

CHAPTER 5 .... **132**

BITTERS FOR IMMUNE HEALTH 132

    Recipe for Immune-Boosting Bitters *133*

HERBS 134

    Get the Energy Combo *135*

WHY PLANTS ARE CRUCIAL TO YOUR IMMUNE SYSTEM CAPABILITY 141

    Blueberries *143*

    Turmeric *144*

    Cordyceps *145*

    Andrographis *146*

    Mushrooms *148*

    Garlic *149*

    Black and Green Tea Extract *150*

    Broccoli Sprouts *151*

    Chinese Skullcap *152*

- *Japanese Knotweed* 153
- *Ginger* 154
- IMPORTANT STEPS TO MAKE IT WORK 154

CHAPTER 6 157

- HEALTHY MINERALS AND VITAMINS 157
  - *Vitamin A* 157
  - *Vitamin C* 158
  - *Vitamin D* 158
  - *Vitamin E* 158
  - *Folate/Folic Acid* 159
  - *Iron* 159
  - *Selenium* 160
  - *Zinc* 160
- FROZEN IS OKAY 161
- IMMUNE BOOSTERS 161
  - *Poultry* 162
  - *Almonds* 163
  - *Mushrooms* 164
  - *Garlic* 165
  - *Citrus Fruits* 166
  - *Pomegranates* 168
  - *Lemons and Zinc* 170
- ORANGE PROBIOTIC IMMUNITY BOOSTING SMOOTHIES 172
  - *Ingredients for Smoothie* 173
- SMOOTHIE TIPS FOR CANCER PATIENTS 177
  - *Focus on Fruit* 177
  - *Include Veggies* 179
  - *Then add Protein.* 179
  - *Pour in a few Liquids.* 180
  - *Give it Improvement.* 181
  - *Try these Mixes.* 182

CHAPTER 7 184

vi

IMMUNE-BOOSTING RECIPES	184
California Salmon	*185*
Chicken Noodle Soup	*186*
Superfood Salad	*188*
Citrus Glazed Roasted Carrots	*189*
Broccoli Rabe and Kale Harvest Salad	*191*
Tuscan Broccoli-Tomato Tarts	*194*
Applewood Smoked Salmon with Warm Potato-Apple Salad and Ale Dressing	*195*
Gingered Carrot-Orange Soup	*198*
Grilled Salmon with Mediterranean Salsa	*199*
Healthy Potato, Spinach, & Pumpkin Seed Hash	*201*
Blueberry Orange and Almond Pancakes With Orange Maple Glaze	*204*
Indian-Spiced Tomato and Black Bean Soup	*206*
Foil-Baked Cod with Oranges, Scallions, and Ginger	*207*
Jerk Shrimp and Citrus Salad	*209*
Tomatillos	*211*
Chicken with Garlic and Parsley	*212*
Roasted Garlic Kale Hummus	*213*
Roasted Sardines, Lemongrass, and Tomatoes	*215*
Rosemary Citrus-Herb Turkey	*217*
Spaghetti Squash and Zucchini	*218*
Spinach Orange Smoothie Recipe	*219*
Middle Eastern Spiced Cauliflower Soup	*220*
Stir-fried fish with chili, ginger, and eggplants	*221*
Braised Beef with Fire-Roasted Green Chilies	*221*
Spinach gratin	*222*
Crisp Eggplant with sweet-spiced yogurt and Pomegranate	*222*
Soy, Ginger, Cumquat, and Gin Oysters	*222*
Slow-Cooked lamb Kashmir Shanks	*223*
Porridge with Spiced Poached Apple	**223**
Stewed Green Beans with Tomato, Chili, and Cinnamon	*224*
Thai-Style Lemongrass and Chili San Choy Bau	*224*
Celeriac, Potato, and Roast Garlic Soup	*225*

Meyer Lemon, Butter Mushroom, Fennel and Radicchio Salad with Parmesan *225*
Vegetarian Pho with Shitake Mushrooms *226*
Stuffed Sweet Potatoes *226*
Chicken and Spelled Soup *227*

CONCLUSION **228**

RECOMMENDED BOOKS **230**

B O N U S : (F R E E B O O K S) **233**

Copyright © 2021 by Dr. Anna Mike Marla

All rights reserved. No part of this publication may be reproduced, distributed, or transmitted in any form or by any means, including photocopying, recording, or other electronic or mechanical methods, without the prior written permission of the publisher, except in the case of brief quotations embodied in critical reviews and certain other non-commercial uses permitted by copyright law.

FREE BONUS

Books are the best and most efficient way to learn something new, it is our life-blood. Through the power of books, we connect with each other, evolve as a society, and find our purpose.

Join the community of over a million and growing enthusiasts readers committed to the literary life, and be among the first to receive notification when I and several Authors have special deals, giveaway, and also ARC (Advanced Readers Copy) of our book(s), and you'd be pleased to sign up to the **Exclusive List** to get access to your **FREE BONUS**.

Your free books download URL is at the end of this book.

Preface

<u>Did you know a healthy immune system is the body's primary defense against disease and infection?</u>

It is also the body's primary defense against cancer. Your immune system is made up of many different types of white blood cells. Each type is specially designed to fight a certain type of disease or infection.

Most often, your body is fighting an invisible enemy that is trying to kill you. That's why you get sick all the time. In fact, you probably get sick more than you do anything else. When you get sick, your body is trying to give you what it thinks is the best chance it has to fight off the "bad guy" (virus or bacteria).

But the truth is, when your body is fighting an infection, it is actually creating antibodies that are literally "starving" the germs/viruses for nutrients.

That's why many people who get a flu shot every year almost never get the flu. Instead, they get a mild cold that lasts a few days. That's because their bodies are busy creating those "starving" antibodies.

What if you could make it easier on your Immune System?

This is an immune system defense guidebook about how to boost your body's natural defenses. It contains information you may not have considered before, and shows you *how to improve your energy levels, reduce stress, get a better night's sleep, disease fighting capability, vitality and longevity.*

Why Should You Take Boosting of Your Immune System Seriously?

- A weakened or exhausted immune system defense makes you more vulnerable to illness and disease
- Help protect your body against harmful viruses and bacteria that cause colds, the flu and other illnesses.
- Help support a healthy weight so you don't put extra stress on your heart and circulatory system.
- Help increase your energy levels throughout the day.
- Help improve your memory and focus.
- Help cleanse your lymphatic system.
- Help keep your skin healthy and toxin-free.
- A properly nourished, strong immune system gives you the best chance of staying healthy and fighting off infections

- The foods you eat have a direct effect on the strength and activity of your immune system
- An unhealthy immune system can lead to chronic fatigue, depression, weight gain, and many other health problems
- When you have a strong immune system, you have the energy to fight off colds and the flu
- Your white blood cells, antibodies, and phagocytes (specialized cells that ingest and destroy unwanted invaders) work better, which means they attack cancer cells, HIV, and other diseases
- Your body makes antibody "swipe files" that contain information on what it has previously encountered. If you come across a microbe or virus you have never before seen, your immune system will create a "virtual" immunity to it.
- Your immune system is able to distinguish between "friend" and "foe". This means that if you are fighting an infection, your body treats the invader as a threat, and works to get rid of it.

...and many more!

This immune system booster book suitable for kids and adults is the body's defense against viruses, bacteria, fungi (mold), and certain types of cancer. *It works in conjunction with your nervous system, your lymphatic system, and your cardiovascular system*. Basically, it's everything working together to keep you healthy. When your defenses are strong, you are less likely to fall prey to viruses, bacteria, and other infections.

Introduction

There are various healthy methods to strengthen your disease-fighting ability (immune system).

Your first type of defense is to choose a healthy lifestyle. Following through on general good-health guidelines may be the single best step you can take towards boosting your disease-fighting ability naturally.

It will also ensure that your disease-fighting ability is strong and healthy. All of the body, including your disease fighting capability, works better when protected from environmental attacks and bolstered by healthy-living strategies such as these:

- Don't smoke,
- Eat a diet rich in fruits & vegetables,
- Exercise regularly,
- Maintain a healthy weight,
- If you drink alcohol; ensure you drink moderately,
- Get adequate sleep,
- Take steps to avoid infection, such as washing the hands frequently and cooking meats thoroughly,

- Make an effort to minimize stress, and Boost immunity the healthy way.

Many products on store shelves claim to improve or boost immunity. However, the idea of boosting immunity makes little sense scientifically. Boosting the number of cells in your immune cells or others is not necessarily a very important thing. For instance, athletes who take part in "blood doping", pumping blood to their systems to improve their quantity of blood cells and improve their performance, risking the chance of stroke.

Attempting to increase the cells of your immune system is particularly complicated because there are a wide variety of cell types in the disease-fighting capability that react to a wide variety of microbes in different ways.

Which cells would you boost, and also to what number? Till now, scientists have no clue what the answer could be. What's known is the fact that the body is continually generating immune cells. Certainly, it produces a lot of lymphocytes than it could use. The excess cells remove themselves through a natural procedure for cell death called apoptosis, some before they see any action; some after they have been able to fight against the external bodies wanting to gain entry into the body.

Nobody knows how many cells or what the best combination of cells the disease fighting capability require to function at its optimum level.
The best thing to do is to give the body the best chance to fight infection and illness.

Perhaps you are down with a cold – you should take *vitamin C and zinc*, maybe even sip some warm chicken noodle soup. Taking time to recover can be important to help your immune system do its work, says H. James Wedner, an allergist at Washington University and Barnes-Jewish Hospital in St. Louis.

In addition, when you are frequently fighting illnesses, experts say it's important you meet with a health provider who can see whether an underlying medical cause, including an immunodeficiency, is at fault. Taking such precautions is especially crucial now, with public health authorities scrambling to support the coronavirus pandemic. Individuals who have underlying medical conditions - such as <u>cardiovascular disease, lung disease, or diabetes</u> - are particularly susceptible to coronavirus, experts say. Nevertheless, you should not wait until you're sick to improve your disease-fighting capability.

As we age, our disease fighting ability becomes reduced, which considerably leads to more infections including cancer. As the life span in developed countries has increased, so does the incidence of age-related conditions.

Although some people age healthily, the outcome of several studies in the research weighed against younger people. Older people are more likely to contract infectious diseases and, more importantly, they are more prone to die from this range of diseases. Respiratory infections, influenza, the **COVID-19** virus, and particularly pneumonia are one of the causes of death in people who are above the age of 65 across the world.

No one can explain this; however, many scientists discover that this increased risk is related to a reduction in T cells, possibly from your thymus atrophying with age and the production of fewer T cells to fight off infection.

Whether this reduction in thymus function explains the drop in T cells or whether other changes are likely involved, it is not fully understood.

Other needs in the bone marrow become less efficient at producing the stem cells that provide an increase in the cells in the immune system.

A decrease in immune reactions to infections continues to be demonstrated by older people's responses to vaccines. For instance, studies of influenza vaccines show that for people above the age of 65, the vaccine is less effective in comparison to healthy children (above the age of 2). But regardless of the decrease in efficacy, vaccinations for influenza and S. Pneumoniae have significantly lowered the rates of sickness and death in the elderly in comparison to no vaccination.

Chapter 1
The Human Immune System

The Human immune system capability is huge. It is the second largest after your liver. But since it spreads throughout the body, you are most likely aware of it in a little way. Lymph nodes are everywhere. The disease-fighting capability offers its organs, just like the thymus and the spleen. Its cells permeate the bloodstream. Your tonsils and adenoids and appendix are all areas of defense mechanisms, and so may be the inside of your bones! Briefly, we'll take a look at several components of the disease fighting capability, the way they work, and how they fit together.

Function of the Immune System

You have the immune system in the body for only one reason. In its absence, the body will be a delightful place for microorganisms like bacteria, viruses, fungi, and parasites to reside and raise their own families. Your body is usually warm, wet, and chock filled with the nutrients microbes it needs to survive and reproduce its own kind.

Compare that with how microbes in other areas are known to live: e.g. boiling sulfur vents in the bottom of the ocean, or under the frozen Arctic tundra. You shouldn't expect gratitude from the microbes that have made your body their home. Almost all of them don't care what happens to you. A few of them can make you very sick. Some can kill you, which can hinder what nature has organized for you to survive and reproduce your kind.

How the Immune System Functions

Microbes have been around a long time before humans. Initially, all forms of life on the planet consisted of only a single cell, now there are many of them, like the bacteria and the fungi, which remain as single cells.

It is not certain when the single-cell microbes evolved into more technical multi-celled plants and animals, it wasn't a long time before some of the more active ones who stayed behind stopped surviving in the hostile environment provided by the still young earth and replaced themselves with their multicellular descendants.

To do this, complex organisms had to build up systems to safeguard themselves. Fortunately for all of us, they did! And incidentally, humans are not in any way unique in having immune systems. Every multicellular organism upon this planet, both plant and animal, faced the same problem and had to build some kind of microbial immune system.

The microbes didn't just relax and allow larger animals and plants to build defense systems they cannot penetrate and take advantage of. The history of the evolution of larger plants and animals is to a large extent, the story of the co-evolution of larger organisms with their microbial enemies. For every defense strategy developed by multicellular organisms against microbes, the microbes developed counter-strategies to evade them. Subsequently, their hosts are forced to build up a new body defense mechanism or be destroyed.

Microbes have one distinct advantage that is necessary for the continuity of the human race: the speed of reproduction. One of the dominant themes in evolution is size. Over evolutionary time, animals generally became bigger. There are several known reasons for this, but probably one of the most obvious is that the bigger you are the higher the chances of being a predator instead of a prey. But of course, the bigger you are, the longer time it takes to put you together from scratch. A bacterium, if it can stay warm and get enough to feed on, can reproduce itself in less than one hour. We have a dozen years roughly at minimum.

The important reason is the fact that evolutionary changes, in reaction to environmental threats like extinction, emanate from changes within an evolving organism's **DNA** mutations in its genes that make it a reproductive advantage over its siblings and cousins, and aunts. And the major way to obtain these mutations is necessary when **DNA** is reproduced through the generation of offspring.

Whenever a cell divides, the DNA in the "parent" cell has to be copied to create DNA for "daughter" cells. This copying is fairly precise; it must be when the offspring is likely to be a complete replica of the parent. Or else, it isn't precise. Mistakes are made during the copying of DNA. Many of these copy errors are edited out.

However, the editing process can be imperfect, and a small number of changes creep into DNA and genes. These slight variations in genes between generations provide the raw stuff of evolution and natural selection. What does this have to do with your competition for dominance and survival, versus submission and death, between single-cell microbes and more technical organisms such as ourselves?

Don't microbes help to make mistakes, too?
Yes, but think about this. In case a fertilized human egg and a bacterium enter into a race to find out who will make more cells, within the first three days of the nine months it requires to produce a newborn human, the bacterium which, remember, can double every half hour or so would have been able to replicate itself to equal the number of humans now alive on the face of the earth!

Of course, this might never happen, as the bacterium and its descendants could never get enough food to keep the reproductive process going.
But you begin to see the problem. Microbes can generate the genetic adjustments that drive their evolution trillions

of times faster than humans. So larger organisms like us had to build up a repertoire of tricks to keep using the microbes' incredible reproductive (and mutational) pace.

The kind of immune systems we have which came with evolutionary existence using the vertebrates (fish, amphibians, reptiles, birds, and mammals like us), cannot recognize and destroy not only every microbe that currently exists but also any microbe that may ever evolve anytime soon, whether we have seen anything like it before or not.

We'll see how we ingenious mammals do that in the next chapter, however, now let's a take look at the way the immune system evolved in our bodies.

Human Immune System Make up

We stated earlier that even the first multicellular animals and plants on earth had some kind of immune system to defend themselves against the invasion of microbial predators.

As living things became more complex, so did their body's defense mechanism. A few of these mechanisms were successful enough to have been transferred into humans. They are a kind of an integral part of our defenses against microbes called *innate immunity*. This means that your disease fighting capability contains some components which have been around for a billion years or even more, furthermore to the recent mechanisms only found in invertebrates.

For quite some time, scientists assumed that innate immunity was only a quaint reminder of a youthful period and a cruder immune system that is no longer essential to our survival. Nothing can be further from reality. We cannot survive without it. The issue is it is no longer effective to protect us completely.

The Bone Marrow

A good place to start a description of the mammalian immune system is the bone marrow. This is the pale yellowish-white, jelly-like substance at the center of all bones in the body. The function of the bone marrow is to oversee the multiplication of all or any of the cells within the blood.

Many of these are _red blood cells_ ("**erythrocytes**"), which carry oxygen and present blood in its color but scattered among these red blood cells in our bodies are the _white blood cells_ ("**leukocytes**"), which are the foot soldiers of the immune system.

The only real job of white blood cells is to prevent invasion by microbial predators. All red blood cells are alike, but what we refer to collectively as white blood cells is a variety of many types of white cells, each having a different and important immune function.

Both red and white blood cells originate from something called a **bone marrow stem cell**. The state name of the stem cell is the hematopoietic stem cell, meaning a stem cell that provides rise to cells within the blood.

The stem cells on the bone marrow usually do not have the characteristics of mature blood cells, but something intriguing happens to stem cells if they are triggered to separate. Normally, whenever a cell divides, it produces two identical daughter copies of itself. However when stem cells split, they do so asymmetrically, they produce one daughter that's an exact copy of themselves and another that could be ready to take off through the stem cell parent and live off its self.

In the situation of *hematopoietic stem cells*, one daughter can be an exact copy of the stem cell, and the other daughter will be a cell that moves down a pathway, hence, causing the production of one of the blood cell types - a red cell, or one of the numerous types of white cells we'll meet shortly.

The *hematopoietic stem cell* is the critical cell in a bone marrow transplant. It could bring about every cell in the blood, but these transplants can be quite dangerous.

The Thymus

The thymus is a glandular organ that lays above the heart. In gourmet kitchens all over the world, the thymus from calves and lambs can, with appropriate skill, be converted into something called sweetbreads.

However, in the body, it's the place for the development of a special immune cell called a **T cell**, the "T" reflecting its thymic origin. These cells arise from stem cells in the bone marrow; however, they leave the bone marrow through the blood before they are fully mature and prepared to protect the body system against microbial invaders. The time of thymic maturation is especially important since it is where T cells learn what is in the body and what's not. Failure to create this distinction can result in the disease-fighting capability turning against self, which results in autoimmunity.

The thymus reaches its maximum size during adolescence and declines gradually thereafter.

Lymphocytes

Among the types of white blood cells produced by the bone marrow stem cells are the lymphocytes. There are two major subsets of lymphocytes: **T cells and B cells**.

T cells, as we've simply seen, get their name from the fact that they need to go through the thymus to complete their maturation. The intense selection they undergo in the thymus leads to the death of at least 90% of the T cells due to stem cells in the bone marrow. They are presumably the T cells that may potentially react with self components. B cells arise in and complete their entire maturation in the bone marrow.

The work of B cells is to produce a blood protein called an **antibody,** *which hunts down and helps to destroy foreign invaders swimming around in body fluids.* **T cells** do not produce antibodies. Rather, they promote an itchy, painful process called inflammation, which serves as a powerful defense against a variety of microbial invaders.

T cells also support B cells in making antibodies. As we will have, one highly specialized T cell, called a killer T cell, can look for and physically destroy cells in the body determined to harbor viruses or other intracellular parasites.

There are a variety of other key players in the white cell repertoire that play crucial roles in our reaction to foreign invaders, but rather than describe all of them here, we can examine them when we encounter them in the real-life situations they were made to cope with.

<u>Both lymphocytes we just examined - T and B cells-</u> provide one of the most important distinctions between the

immune systems of vertebrates like us and the immune defense systems of animals that came earlier.

They give us using a spectacularly precise, highly nuanced, and intensely effective immune system that earthworms could only dream of.

Lymph Nodes and Spleen

When T cells and B cells reach full maturity, they leave the thymus and bone marrow, respectively, and migrate to take up residence in the lymph nodes and spleen. You only have one spleen, a big red organ close to the stomach, but you can have a huge selection of small lymph nodes scattered throughout the entire body.

These structures are not only tiny sacs full of cells, however, but lymph nodes also have a strict internal structure that is replicated in most nodes. B cells are located mostly in the external (*cortex*) region of every node; T cells are found in a region called the **paracortex**. As blood and lymph go through these structures, the substances they are carrying are trapped there and examined. Potential useful materials will also be taken to lymph nodes from around your body by a particular scavenging cell called a ***dendritic cell***.

All this is examined closely by **T and B cells**. Whatever is *"self"* is permitted to pass through. Anything that is *"not-self"* triggers some alarms and sets an immune response in motion, activating *T cells and B cells* that recognize the offending antigen as foreign. B cells, once activated, start to create and secrete the protein called an ***antibody***, which we will discuss at length in the next two chapters.

The activated T cells leave the lymph nodes, going on patrol in the body to search out the source of the problem. When they identify it, they organize an attack that results in clearing the offending material from the body.

The spleen has several functions. One of these is to eliminate dead and dying red cells in the blood and recover the iron from the hemoglobin they carry. But parts of the spleen also function as a huge lymph node and trap foreign material for inspection by resident *T and B cells*.

What is the Lymph?

The blood does more than carry red and white blood cells around the body. Besides, it carries digested food and oxygen to all or any of the body's tissues. These foods are dissolved in the liquid part with the blood (plasma) and so are unloaded through the tiny arteries called the *capillaries*. The red cells unload their oxygen and tighten the skin, and the foods are absorbed by cells that are close by, which discharge waste material from previous meals into nearby cell-bathing fluids.

One of the ways the flow of liquid from blood to tissue would quickly dry out circulation and the body tissues is a <u>*soggy, bloated mess*</u>. The body's approach to the delivery of food and oxygen creates a huge plumbing problem, which is solved by creating a lymphatic drainage system. Where there are capillaries in the body (and that's everywhere), you will find a group of drains and drainpipes called *lymphatic sinuses and lymphatic vessels*.

They are much like veins, although somewhat more fragile. They drain the surplus fluid from around cells and tissues and push it back to the blood circulation. Whereas arteries split up into smaller and smaller branches and finally become capillaries, the lymphatic vessels start tiny and then merge into a group of major trunks that eventually empty lymph fluid back to the bloodstream at the veins on the neck. Aside from its task to maintain the plumbing in the body, mammals depend on the lymphatic draining system to defend and protect their immune system.

It is with the spread of the lymphatic network that these lymph nodes are stationed. Remember, most of the things that travel through the blood result in lymphatic circulation; therefore the various lymphatic branches and trunks are ideal places to monitor what goes on in the body.

The lymph nodes are also served by arteries, so it can be difficult for anything traveling around the body in either blood or lymph to escape surveillance in the lymph nodes.

The spleen, while not receiving lymph fluids, nonetheless acts as a highly effective filter for foreign materials in the blood.

When you have a cut or other wound, microbes, and other potentially harmful material, can cross into tissue spaces, where they can be quickly swept into the general lymphatic traffic and trickle through downstream lymph nodes.

As regards cancer, cells escaping from a tumor into surrounding tissue fluids can also be trapped in a nearby lymph node. That's the reason for many cancers. Doctors collect nearby surrounding lymph nodes for examination with a pathologist. The existence or lack of cancer cells in these nodes is an essential aspect of planning treatment strategies.

Ways to Keep the Immune System Healthy

Many important healthy lifestyle habits can help to keep your immune system active to resist sickness and infections. The body (together with your immune system) works on the fuel you put into it. That's why eating good food, along with having a healthy diet routine is indeed important.

Simply put, it is your immune system's responsibility to guard the body against illness and disease. The complex system comprises of cells in the skin layer, blood, bone marrow, tissues, and organs that - when working as they ought to - protect the body against potentially harmful pathogens (like bacteria and viruses), and limit damage from non-infectious agents (like sunburn or cancer), according to the National Institutes of Health (**NIH**).

Think about the immune system as an orchestra. To have the best performance, you want every instrument and every musician in the orchestra to perform at its best. You won't want one musician performing on double speed or one instrument, suddenly producing sound at twice the quantity it usually does. You will want every part of the orchestra to perform exactly according to plan.

The same applies to the immune system. To best protect the body from harm, every part of the immune system must work exactly according to plan.
The simplest way to do this is to daily adopt healthy habits that can strengthen your immune system.
We shall begin to discuss each of the important ways of keeping a healthy immune system.

Eat a Healthy Diet Plan

The nutrients you get from food, specifically, *plant-based foods like fruits, vegetables, herbs, and spices* are crucial to maintaining your disease fighting capability and to also help it function properly. Many plant-based foods also have antiviral and antimicrobial homes that help us to fight off infections.

For instance, research implies that spices like *clove, oregano, thyme, cinnamon, and cumin contain antiviral and antimicrobial properties* that prevent the growth of food-spoiling bacteria like Bacillus subtilis and Pseudomonas fluorescens, harmful fungi like Aspergillus flavus, and antibiotic-resistant microorganisms like Staphylococcus aureus, according to an assessment posted in June 2017 in the International Journal of Molecular Sciences.

Furthermore, the *zinc, folate, iron, selenium, copper, and vitamins A, C, E, B6, and B12* you get from the meals you eat are the nutrients your immune system will need to perform its duty, according to the Academy of Nutrition and Dietetics. Each one plays a distinctive role in supporting immune function.

Research suggests, for instance, that vitamin C deficiency can increase the probability of infection, according to an assessment published in November 2017 in Nutrients. Our anatomies do not produce this essential, water-soluble vitamin independently, so we have to obtain it through foods (such as citric fruits, kiwis, and many cruciferous vegetables). You can get 95 milligrams (mg) or 106 percent from the everyday vitamin C you will need by eating a half-cup of red pepper, according to the NIH.

Protein is crucial for immune health. The proteins in protein-based food help to build and maintain immune cells, and skimping upon this macronutrient can reduce your body's ability to fight infections. In a single study published in February 2013 in the Journal of Infectious Diseases, mice that ate a diet plan comprising only 2 percent protein were more severely affected by flu than mice that ate a *"normal protein"* diet with 18 percent protein. But once researchers started feeding the first group a *"normal protein"* diet, the mice was able to eliminate the virus.

With regards to an eating plan that supports good immune health, concentrate on incorporating more plants and plant-based foods. *Add fruits and veggies to soups and stews, smoothies, and salads, or eat them as snacks.*
<u>Carrots, broccoli, spinach, red bell peppers, apricots, citrus fruits (such as oranges, grapefruit, tangerines), and strawberries</u> are all great sources of vitamins A and C,

while *seeds and nuts* will provide protein, vitamin E, and zinc, according to the Academy of Nutrition and Dietetics.

Other resources of protein and zinc include seafood, lean meat, and poultry, according to the Academy of Nutrition and Dietetics.

Get a lot of Quality Sleep

The body heals and regenerates when you sleep, building adequate sleep is crucial for a healthy immune response. More specifically, *sleep is a period when your body produces and distributes important immune cells like* **cytokines** *(a kind of protein that may either fight or promote inflammation), T cells (a kind of white blood cell that regulates immune response), and interleukin 12 (a pro-inflammatory cytokine), according to some review published in Pflugers Archiv European Journal of Physiology.*

Whenever you don't get enough sleep, your immune system might not perform these functions well, hereby, placing it in a vulnerable position to defend the body against harmful invaders and opening you up to the possibility of being sick.

One report released in July-August 2017 on the problem of Behavioral Sleep Medicine shows that; compared with healthy young adults who did not have sleep problems, otherwise healthy young adults with insomnia were more susceptible to flu even after getting vaccinated.

Sleep deprivation also increases cortisol levels, which is also bad for immune function. "Our disease fighting capability wears down because of this, and we generally have (fewer) reserves to fight off or get over an illness."

The National Sleep Foundation recommends all adults reach at least seven hours of sleep per night to optimize health.

To ensure you get quality sleep, prioritize good sleep hygiene: Switch off the electronics at least 2 to 3 hours before bed, and avoid violent or stressful books or conversations.

With regards to Alcohol, Practice Moderation

Drinking too much alcohol can be associated with a variety of negative health effects, including a weak system. Once you consume alcohol excessively, the body becomes busy trying to detoxify itself to work with normal immune system function.

According to an assessment published in the journal Alcohol Research in 2015, high amounts of alcohol can weaken your body's ability to fight infection and decelerate your recovery period. Because of this, people who drink excessive amounts of alcohol are prone to *pneumonia, acute respiratory distress syndrome, alcoholic liver disease, and certain cancers*, based on the same review.

If you don't drink, don't start. If you drink occasionally, limit your alcohol intake to 1 drink (equal to a 4-ounce glass of wine) per day if you're a female, and two drinks each day if you're a male, as recommended by the NIH.

Keep Stress in Check

According to a study published in October 2015 problem of Current Opinion in Mindset, *long-term stress leads to chronically elevated degrees of the steroid hormone cortisol.* The body relies on hormones like ***cortisol*** during short-term bouts of stress (when your body goes into a "fight-or-flight" response); cortisol plays a beneficial role in actually preventing the immune system from responding before the stressful event is over (so your body can react to the immediate stressor). But when cortisol levels are constantly high, it blocks the immune system from kicking into gear and to do its job by protecting the body against potential threats from germs like viruses and bacteria.

<u>There are different effective stress-reduction techniques; the main element is to discover what works for you.</u> "I love to give my patients options," says Ben Kaplan, MD, an internal medicine doctor at Orlando Health Medical Group Internal Medicine in Florida.

He recommends meditation *(apps like Headspace and Calm can help)*, writing, and any activity that you enjoy (such as fishing, playing golf, or drawing). Try to do at least one stress-reducing activity every day.

Are you short on time?

Start small at intervals, set five (5) minutes aside for fun each day, and go ahead to increase it when you can.

Keep Symptoms of Chronic Conditions in Order

Chronic conditions like *asthma, cardiovascular disease, and diabetes* make a difference in the immune system and increase the risk of infections.

For instance, when people who have type 2 diabetes don't manage their blood sugar levels properly, this can lead to a chronic, low-grade inflammatory response that weakens the body's immune system, according to an October 2019 review in Current Diabetes Reviews.

Similarly, people who have asthma tend to be more vulnerable to catching and dying from the flu and frequently experience worse flu and asthma symptoms due to *chlamydia*, according to a report published in the July 2017 issue of the Journal of Allergy and Clinical Immunology.

Coping with a chronic condition can be likened to wanting to drive a vehicle that has only three tires. "In case you get sick via a virus, it's going to take more effort for your body to recuperate".

If you manage your chronic situations well, you'll release more reserves to help the body fight off infection. So ensure to stick to the top of any medications, doctor visits, and healthy habits that can keep your symptoms away. Your immune system will be grateful for doing so.

Let's talk about food that will help boost your immune system function.

Don't Smoke Cigars

Like alcohol, using tobacco can also affect immune health. "Anything that is a toxin can compromise your disease-fighting ability,".

Specifically, the chemicals released by tobacco smoke carbon monoxide, nicotine, nitrogen oxides, and cadmium can hinder the growth and function of immune cells, like cytokines, T cells, and B cells, according to a November 2016 review in Oncotarget.

Smoking also worsens viral and microbe infections (especially those of the lungs, like pneumonia, flu, and tuberculosis), post-surgical infections, and arthritis rheumatoid (an autoimmune disease where the disease fighting capability attacks the joints), according to the CDC.

"Don't smoke,". And avoid second-hand smoking whenever you can.

If you currently smoke, there are different resources open to help you combat your addiction, which includes counseling, nicotine replacement products, prescription non-nicotine medications, and behavioral therapy, according to the CDC.

Exercise Regularly (Outdoors, When Possible)

Regular physical exercise lowers your chance of developing chronic diseases (like *obesity, type 2 diabetes, and cardiovascular disease*), and also viral and transmissions, according to a review in Frontiers in Immunology in April 2018.

Exercise also increases the release of endorphins (several hormones that decrease pain and create feelings of pleasure) making it a terrific way to manage stress. "Since stress negatively affects our disease fighting capability, this is another way exercise can improve immune response.

And while there is evidence that lengthy or intense exercise sessions may suppress the disease-fighting capability, it makes you even more vulnerable to illness and infection within the hours immediately after your workout, the data on that question is contradictory, according to the same Frontiers in Immunology review.

And there is a wealth of epidemiological evidence (studies that followed human behavior and outcomes) showing that more active people generally tend to have lower incidences of both acute illnesses (like infections) and chronic ones (like cancer, and type 2 diabetes). Studies that have looked at how exercise affects the body on a cellular level suggest that bouts of physical activity can make your immune system more active by distributing immune cells throughout your body to look for damaged or infected cells, according to a 2018 report.

At least, try to meet up with the exercise guidelines outlined by the Centers for Disease Control and Prevention (CDC). Adults ought to be getting at least 150 minutes (2 to 5 hours) of moderate-intensity aerobic fitness exercise (like walking, jogging, or cycling) or 75 minutes (1 hour and quarter-hour) of high-intensity aerobic fitness exercise (like running) every week. You should also be doing strength training at least twice a week.

Note: *More activity is linked to even more health benefits, so aim high.*

For more disease-fighting capability benefits, I suggest taking your exercise outside. Hanging out among natural scenery has been shown to aid mood, lower blood pressure, reduce inflammation, and support immune health.

Sunshine also boosts vitamin D in the body, which plays an integral role in immune health too.

Prepare to Strengthen Your Immune System

Based on the recent coronavirus (**COVID-19**) outbreak, many people are concerned about staying healthy and maintaining a healthy defense mechanism. Doing so will benefit the body and increase your defenses against viruses, bacteria, and other pathogens. In the slides below, we will discuss the best immunity boosting ideas to assist you and your body stay strong to fight off infections.

Your Social Life can Make You Stronger

Increasing evidence from many reports suggests loneliness and social isolation have become detrimental to health. In a single study, people that have the strongest social relationships are likely to live longer than those that have poor social connections.

There are several methods to develop and strengthen social ties.

- Grab the telephone and call friends regularly.
- Make plans to hang out together.
- Volunteer for any cause you genuinely believe in.
- Join a class or join an organization related to an interest or hobby you have.
- Keep up with old friends and make new ones to strengthen and expand your social circle.

Regular Sex is Helpful

In a report of university students, those that had sex a few times weekly had the best levels of **immunoglobulin A (IgA)** in their saliva.

IgA is an immune molecule that protects us against illnesses like the common cold. Students who had sex a couple of times each week had more salivary IgA than students who have not been sexually active, infrequently sexually active (less than once a week), or who had been very sexually active (three or more times weekly).

Enjoying sex up to a couple of times weekly seems to be the sweet spot for promoting optimal IgA levels.

Processed Foods Diet deprive the Body of Nutrients

Processed foods include candy, soda, junk foods, and snacks. They contain zero calories and do not provide the body with vitamins, nutrients, or fiber. They often also contain chemicals and preservatives that are not good for the body.

When you eat processed foods rather than foods in their natural, unprocessed form, the body is deprived of nutrients and vitamins that it requires to thrive.

Avoid processed foods, and embrace more fruits, vegetables, lean meat, healthy fats, and whole grains to give the body and immune system everything they need to function at their best. *Optimize your dietary habits to support your health.*

Optimize Your Diet for Optimal Immune Function

Antioxidants are compounds in fruits & vegetables that drive back free radicals. Free radicals may damage DNA and other cell components. Fruits & vegetables in several colors supply the best mixture of protective antioxidants to improve general health and immunity.

<u>Eat leafy greens, watermelon, carrots, berries, broccoli, oranges, kiwi, cantaloupe, and other colorful produce to provide your cells and disease-fighting capability with all the natural protection they need to operate optimally.</u>

Homemade chicken soup with carrots, celery, and other veggies can also be a boon to your immune system.

Fight Disease with Laughter.

Can laughter increase your disease-fighting capability? The results of some studies suggest it could. In a report of healthy males, watching a funny movie boosted natural killer cell activity while watching an emotionally neutral movie didn't boost the activity of the disease fighting capability. While more research is essential to determine a conclusive link between laughter and improved immunity, go on, and have a good chuckle. Belly laughs feel good. They can't injure and they might support your disease fighting capability and also decrease the probability of illness.

Multivitamin Can Help

Some experts think that taking multivitamins daily might help to ensure you're meeting your minimum daily requirement of essential nutrients.

Vitamins that are crucial for immune function include **Vitamins A, C, D, and E. Zinc, selenium, and**

magnesium are minerals that your disease-fighting capability needs to function at its best.

These minerals are crucial for the functioning of numerous enzyme reactions in the body. Your immune system and body can't function at their best without the basic building blocks they need to work properly.

Pets are a Boon to Immunity

Results of studies also show that owners have lower blood pressure and cholesterol levels in comparison to those who do not own pets. Owners had lower cholesterol and triglycerides in comparison to non-pet owners.

This might imply higher overall heart health and reduced risk of heart problems. Pet owners may enjoy improved heart health simply because they are more likely to engage in physical activity because they walk their dogs regularly. Pet ownership in childhood is linked to decreased susceptibility to allergies.

Stress

Chronic stress depresses the disease-fighting capability and escalates the risk of various kinds of illnesses. It increases the number of hormones called catecholamines. Being overtaken by stress leads to increased levels of suppressor T cells, which suppress the disease-fighting capability. When this part of the disease fighting capability is impaired, you tend to be more vulnerable to viral illnesses, including respiratory conditions like *colds, flu, and the novel coronavirus infection.*

Stress leads to the release of *histamine*, a molecule involved in allergies - combat stress with techniques like *deep breathing, meditation, exercise, and relaxation.*

Be Positive to Improve Immune Response

Expect good stuff, and your disease-fighting capability will follow. Research on law students discovered that their immune systems were stronger whenever they felt optimistic.

- Be optimistic about meeting your needs.
- Try to see the glass as half full, not half empty.
- Practice gratitude and think about at least three things that you will be grateful for every day.

Imagine the best outcome for situations, even difficult ones. You may not always be able to control events around you, but you can constantly decide how to respond to them. Respond with a sound attitude to increase the chances of the best outcome and to strengthen your immunity.

Chapter 2

Natural Ways to Boost the Immune System

A healthy disease-fighting capability reduces your potential for viral infection and flu. With these natural ways to boost the immune system, you can have a healthy disease-fighting capability.

During flu or viral season, a lot of your friends might fall sick easily; however, many will stand tall during this period even when everyone in their home is down with the flu.

Have you ever wondered how many people get sick often, and how some people are prone to catching a cold or viral infection? It's all about the body's immune system.

<u>The immune system is the first line of defense in the body against any foreign microorganism entering the body.</u>

The stronger your immune system, the lesser your chances of falling sick. *But then, having a strong immune system doesn't make you invincible.*

With a little change in what you eat and your routine, you can ensure that your immune system is strong enough to protect you against virus infection. From sleeping for eight hours to walking in sunlight to eating a balanced diet, the methods are simple; however, they are really helpful if followed. Follow them and witness the change in your body's ability to fight illness.

Lessen Your Stress Levels

Chronic stress suppresses the immune response of your body by releasing the hormone cortisol. Cortisol inhibits the T-cells (a particular white blood cell) to replicate and receive signals from your body. Cortisol also reduces the antibody secretory **IgA**, which lines the gut and respiratory system, which is the first line of defense against pathogens.

To keep your stress in check, *practice yoga, meditation, or deep breathing daily.*

Reduce your Alcohol Intake.

Numerous researches show that excess alcohol intake can affect the immune system and pathway in a complicated manner. However, moderate consumption of alcohol is a good idea for the overall health of the body.

Ensure You Get Your A-B-C-D-Es

The adage, "an apple a day keeps the doctor away" can be true as the consumption of vitamins can boost your immune system.

Vitamin A, B6, C, D, and E can help to boost the strength of the immune system. Vitamin C is the biggest booster of all, and lack of it can cause several diseases, including Scurvy. You can get Vitamin C from citrus fruits like Orange, Grapefruit, Spinach, and Strawberries. You can take multivitamin supplements from your doctor; however, natural intake through food is the best way.

Try Colostrum

Colostrum is described as the first milk from nursing mammals. The benefit of being breastfed is the intake of protective antibodies you get from your mother. These antibodies help you to fight through the early years of your life. These antibodies are the reason why children that are breastfed are healthier and are less likely to catch a cold or be prone to allergies.

We can harness the antibodies of the first milk even when we are adults. In powder form, obtained from cows, goats, and other mammals, these antibodies can be mixed with water, juice, and shakes.

Eat lots of Vegetables

Vegetables, fruits, seeds, and nuts contain nutrients that are crucial for our disease-fighting ability. Eating them regularly improves immunity. For a healthy liver, cruciferous vegetables like Kale, Broccoli, and Cabbage should be included in the daily food diet. A healthy liver oversees the body's natural detoxification process.

Herbs & Supplements

Herbs like AHCC, Echinacea, Elderberry, Andrographis, and Astragalus can help to reduce the duration and severity of illness. Also, using vitamin and mineral supplements provides the necessary nutrients for a strong immune system.

Exercise regularly

Working out frequently continues to be one of the ways to boost the defense mechanisms. Routine workouts mobilize the T cells, a kind of white blood cell which guards your body against infection. However, frequent rigorous workout weakens the immune system, leaving you vulnerable to flu and viral infections.

Get adequate sleep

Insomnia can cause the inflammatory immune reaction to activate, hereby, reducing the experience of T cells in the body. This can weaken the disease-fighting capability and it's response to vaccines. Ensure you rest for 7-8 hours and avoid having an all-nighter. If you will be traveling in various time zones frequently, take 2-3mg of Melatonin to reset the circadian rhythm.

Start to eat Mushrooms

Mushroom is nature's way of wearing down the organic matter to convert them to the fertile soil. Among the healthiest food on earth, mushrooms are rich in essential nutrients and minerals. A number of the mushrooms good for immune systems are A Turkey tail mushroom, Maitake, and Shiitake Mushrooms, Tremella Mushrooms.

Quit smoking

Quit the habit of smoking because not only does it increase the chance of cancer, but it also impairs the disease fighting capability. Smoking is thought to have a poor effect on both adaptive and innate immunity. Also, it can increase the chances of developing harmful pathogenic immune responses. It also reduces the potency of your immune system's defenses.

However, if you desire to continue, you will discover alternatives like the use of nicotine patches or electronic cigarettes that help to stop smoking and make it less harmful.

Step into the sun!

Stepping into sunlight is one of the major ways to aid the production of Vitamin D in our body.

Vitamin D is important for the healthy functioning of the immune system since it helps the body to produce antibodies.

The lack of Vitamin D in the body is known as one of the major causes of respiratory problems.

A quick walk in the sun for 10-15 minutes will ensure that enough Vitamin D is produced in the body.

With these little efforts and tweaks in your daily routine, you can build a healthy immune system. A sound body is not about being healthy outside but also ensuring strong immunity and these 11 natural methods to boost your immunity process can help you achieve the goal of a healthy body.

These steps will reduce the toxins in the body and will provide the needed nutrients which are essential for your health. Keeping a check on the immune system is not only going to keep you safe from falling sick but it will also help you prevent diseases like cancer in the latter half of your life. Also, these natural ways can help you age gracefully.

As regards fighting viruses, everyday precautions such as washing the hands often and avoiding sick people are important. But experts say that boosting your immune system can also give you an advantage in staying healthy. Listed below are five wise steps to increase your to-do list now.

Stay Active

Working out is a robust way to improve your disease-fighting capability, says Mark Moyad, M.D., M.P.H., Jenkins/Pokempner, Director of preventive and alternative medicine at the University of Michigan Infirmary. It causes your antibodies and white blood cells to circulate quicker, which means they might be in a position to detect and zero in on bugs quicker. Being active in this manner also lowers stress hormones, which reduces your chances of falling sick, Moyad adds.

Research shows that the effects of exercise are also highly relevant to fighting against the virus. According to a recently available study published in the British Journal of Sports Medicine, 1,002 people were surveyed, and those that exercised at least five days weekly had almost half the of not being prone to cold compared to those that were more sedentary. If they should catch a cold, they reported less severe symptoms. There can also be an advantage to the sweat being secreted during the exercise: Research shows that simply raising the body temperature can help to kill germs in their tracks.

One vital thing about exercising is to ensure that it is done moderately. "Like many other things, there is a nice spot – exercising without caution can also put a lot of stress on your body, as it depresses your disease fighting capability," explains Moyad. He recommends 30 to 60 minutes of exercise (either vigorous or moderate) most days of the week.

Watch your daily diet

"Eighty percent of the immune system is usually in the gut, so if it is healthy, we have a tendency to be able to fight off infections faster and better," says Yufang Lin, M.D., of the guts for Integrative Medicine on the Cleveland Clinic. "If it is not, our disease fighting capability is weak and more susceptible to overcoming the infection."

Generally, Lin recommends that people focus on the Mediterranean eating style; this means a diet rich in fruits, vegetables, whole grains, and healthy fats, in foods such as fatty fish, nuts, and essential oil. "This eating pattern is saturated in nutrients such as vitamin C, zinc, and other antioxidants proven to reduce inflammation and fight infection," she explains. Adults between the ages of 65 and 79 who followed the Mediterranean eating style, and who go for a daily 400 IU vitamin D supplement for a year, showed small increases in disease-fighting cells such as T cells, according to some 2018 study released in the journal Frontiers in Physiology.

You'll want to limit meat, especially processed and fried foods, which tend to be more inflammatory, Lin adds. "Generally, I would recommend a complete food diet," she says. Also, it's best if you include fermented foods, like yogurt, sauerkraut, miso, and kefir, in your diet. These help to build up the nice bacteria in your gut, which, subsequently, aids a healthy gut and disease-fighting capability, Lin explains.

Stick to the top of the stress

There is a solid link between your immune health and your mental health. "If you are under chronic stress or anxiety, the body produces stress hormones that suppress your disease fighting capability," Moyad says. Research done at Carnegie Mellon University has discovered that stressed people tend to be more vulnerable to developing the normal cold.

In one report, posted in Proceedings from the National Academy of Sciences, 276 healthy adults were subjected to the cold virus, and then monitored in quarantine for five days. Those that had been stressed were more likely to have cytokines, substances that trigger inflammation, and were about doubly likely to become sick. Furthermore, individuals who are stressed are less likely to focus on other healthy habits, like eating right and getting enough sleep, which may affect immunity, Lin adds.

Although you can't avoid stress in your daily life, you can adopt ways to help you to manage it better. A 2012 research, posted in Annals of Internal Medicine, surveyed adults 50 years and older and discovered that those that either did a regular workout routine or performed mindfulness meditation are less inclined to become sick as a result of respiratory infection than subjects within a control group, and even when they fall sick, they only miss out on a few days of work.

Get enough sleep

There is another natural disease-fighting capability booster. "Your disease fighting capability is like your personal computer, it requires intervals of rest so that it doesn't become overheated," Moyad explains. "Sleep reboots the machine."

If you do not get enough sleep, he adds, the body churns out stress hormones like cortisol to keep you awake and alert, which may suppress your disease-fighting capability. People who had a complete eight hours of sleep had higher degrees of T cells than those who slept less, according to a 2019 review.

Try to get at least seven hours of sleep every night, according to a 2015 analysis published in the Sleep journal. The study discovered that people who did so were four times less inclined to come down with a cold than those who slept for less than six hours.

Be Strategic about Supplements

There is no magic herb or vitamin you can pop to automatically prevent a cold, flu, or other viruses. But a 2017 overview of 25 studies, published in the British Medical Journal, discovered that a moderate regular dose of vitamin D can offer protection if you have a deficiency in the vitamin which is provided by the sun, highlights Tod Cooperman, M.D., president and editor in chief of ConsumerLab.com.

The best way to find out if you lack vitamin D is to get your blood levels tested; you ought to be between 20-39 ng/mL (nanograms per milliliter). If you are within that range, and everyday supplement around 600 to 800 IU is okay. If you are low, talk to your doctor about additional supplements as much as 2,000 IU each day. Cooperman advises taking it with meals that contain fats or oils, to improve absorption.

Chapter 3
Foods that Boost and Increase Your Immune System
Elderberry

*"Extracts of **elderberry** have antiviral, anticancer, and anti-inflammatory properties."*

<u>Elderberry</u> is a plant that is being used medicinally for many years. Sambucus nigra, or black elderberry bush, is the variety that is mostly used to create syrup and lozenges. *Extracts of elderberry have antiviral, anticancer, and anti-inflammatory properties.*

Elderberry is saturated with *flavonoids*. People take elderberry syrup as a cure for colds, flu, and bacterial sinus infections.

The medicinal plant functions by reducing swelling in the mucus membranes. Some studies suggest that the juice gotten from elderberry reduces the duration of the flu. If it works for flu infections, it can help your immune system to fight against coronavirus (COVID-19) infection.

Elderberry Drug Interactions

Elderberry has numerous benefits; however, the cure may only work together with some specifically prescribed drugs. Always check with your doctor or pharmacist before adding a new drug or cure to your routine.

Elderberry may not work with the following medications.

Diuretics: *Elderberry is a diuretic*, so taking it with a drug that has a diuretic prescription, increases the effects.

Laxatives: *Elderberry has laxative effects* so it shouldn't be taken with other laxative mediations.

Steroids: Elderberry stimulates the immune system, so it shouldn't be taken with steroids alongside other medications made to suppress the disease-fighting capability of the body. *People who are on immunosuppressive drugs after having undergone organ transplant shouldn't consider elderberry.*

Chemotherapy: Elderberry may hinder chemotherapy and should not be used with it.

Diabetes medications: Elderberry lowers blood sugar levels, so it shouldn't be taken with drugs that treat diabetes.

Theophylline: Elderberry may reduce blood degrees of this drug required to take care of asthma and respiratory conditions.

Mushrooms

Mushrooms are rich in *selenium and vitamin B* like *riboflavin and niacin*, which are necessary for the immune defense to be able to work effectively.

Wondering how you can boost your immune system? Eat more mushrooms. *Mushrooms are also rich in polysaccharides, sugar-like substances that boost immune function.*

Flavorful Fungus

Mushrooms have a savory quality that can improve the flavor of several dishes. Not sure of how to eat mushrooms?

Try the following mouth-watering steps to have these tasty fungi:

- *Sautéing, barbecuing, and roasting can help to draw out the rich, savory flavor of mushrooms.*
- Mushrooms make an excellent addition to scrambled eggs and omelets.
- Toss sliced mushrooms into soups, salads, or lasagna.
- Enjoy Portobello mushroom tops in veggie burgers.
- Stuffed mushrooms make tasty hors d'oeuvres.

Acai Berry

The *acai berry* is rich in anthocyanins that are flavonoid substances that combat oxidative stress in the body and reduce inflammation.

Acai Berry Pulp Benefits

Acai berry is a black-purple fruit that is gotten from the acai berry palm tree in Brazil, Trinidad, and some parts of South USA. The fruit is rich in anthocyanins. These flavonoid substances are very powerful antioxidants. They combat oxidative stress in the body by mopping up free radicals. *Antioxidants* are known for boosting immunity and reducing inflammation in the body. There is never a better time to take pleasure from an acai bowl than now!

Immune-Boosting Fruit

Acai berry pulp is a potent antioxidant and stimulator of the immune system, and researchers are examining it as a potential treatment for all sorts of conditions. Parts of the report include the use of acai in people with:

- ❖ increasing prostate-specific antigen (PSA);
- ❖ Coronary disease and metabolic syndrome;
- ❖ Lower rectum cancer;
- ❖ Constipation, and

Another prospect of studies could include other conditions (for instance, yeast-based infections, Flu, COVID-19).

Oysters

Oysters provide selenium, iron, vitamin C and A, Zinc, and high-quality protein for proper immune function.

Oysters are a nutritional powerhouse from the ocean. One 3-ounce serving of Pacific oysters provides 190% in the daily value of selenium, 45% of the daily value of iron, and 20% on the daily value of vitamin C, all for 140 calories. One 3-ounce serving of oysters contains 16 grams of high-quality protein. The seafood also contains Zinc and Vitamin A. These minerals and vitamins in oysters are crucial for proper immune function.

Ways to Eat Oysters

Many people are familiar with raw oysters served with the half shell, but you will discover that there are several other methods of eating oysters. They include;

- Oysters Rockefeller,
- Oyster Stew,
- Oyster Stuffing,
- Scalloped Oysters, and
- Grilled Oysters.

Watermelon

Watermelon provides the body with vitamins A, C, and B6, nutrients, and compounds like *glutathione* for proper immune functioning.

Watermelon Nutrition

Watermelon is an immune-boosting fruit. One 2-cup serving of watermelon has 270mg of potassium, 30% from the daily value of vitamin A, and 25% of the worth of vitamin C. Calories in watermelon aren't much. One 2-cup serving of watermelon has just 80 calories. *Watermelon also provides vitamin B6 and glutathione.* Your body needs these vitamins, nutrients, and compounds like glutathione for proper immune function.

Five Ways to Eat Watermelon

Watermelon slices is the most typical way to take pleasure from this fruit. Here are some creative ways to eat watermelon.

- Make a fruit salad with watermelon and top it with lemon, honey, and mint dressing.
- Take a tall glass of watermelon strawberry lemonade.
- Snack on arugula watermelon salad topped with feta cheese.
- Enjoy frozen watermelon sorbet.

- Cool-down with watermelon, ginger, lime pops.

Wheat Germ

Wheat germ is rich in B vitamins, zinc, and vitamin E and helps boost nutrition when added to foods.

Wheat germ is the innermost part of the wheat kernel and it is the most nutritious part of the grain. The germ is rich in B vitamins, zinc, and vitamin E. Sprinkle wheat germ with Yogurt or cereal and bring it to some shake.

Wheat germ is a good way to boost the nourishment of cooked goods. Substitute wheat germ for any bit of bleached flour in recipes to get some good extra minerals and vitamins.

What now with Wheat Germ?

A lot of people know that wheat germ makes a very tasty topping when sprinkled on fruit, yogurt, or cereal, but what else can be done with it?

Wheat germ is a versatile food that can be used in several recipes.
- Combine wheat germ, herbs, and spices to make a breaded coating for baked chicken and fish.

- Use wheat germ instead of breadcrumbs in meatloaf and meatballs.
- Sprinkle wheat germ with baked apple crumble and similar desserts.

Yogurt

Yogurt is rich in probiotics and vitamins that can greatly help to boost immunity.

Reasons to like Low-Fat Yogurt

Nourishment guidelines recommend that adults consume three servings of milk products each day. Low-fat yogurt provides 11 grams of protein, 250 calories, and almost 400 mg of calcium per 8-ounce serving. *Low-fat yogurt may also help to meet your daily requirement of vitamin B12, vitamin D, and vitamin B2 (riboflavin).* Adequate quantities of vitamin D, as well as other nutrients, are essential for robust immune function.

Yogurt is rich in probiotics, including Lactobacillus acidophilus, Lactobacillus casei, and Bifidus. These strains boost immune function and can even lessen both the length and severity of colds. Beneficial gut flora is necessary for proper digestion, detoxification, and immune function. Probiotics even lessen eczema symptoms in babies.

Five Ways to Eat Yogurt

A lot of people eat yogurt straight from the cup, but you can find many other methods to enjoy this immune-boosting food.

- Mix yogurt, juice, and a little bit of honey together. Pour into molds and freeze to create yogurt pops.
- Enjoy cucumber salad with yogurt dill dressing.
- Get coleslaw with yogurt rather than mayonnaise.
- Serve fish topped with minted yogurt sauce.
- Use yogurt in creamy soup recipes to give them a tart kick.

Spinach

Spinach contains folate, vitamin A, vitamin C, fiber, magnesium, and iron to improve immune functioning.

- Super Spinach.
- Leafy Green Superfood.

Spinach is rated as a superfood due to the high level of folate, vitamin A, vitamin C, fiber, magnesium, and iron it contains. The nutrients in spinach boost the immune system and provide your body with the necessary nutrients for cell division and DNA repair. Get maximum advantages from spinach by eating it raw or slightly cooked to preserve nutrients.

Think beyond Spinach Salad

Many people are familiar with spinach salad, but how else can spinach be prepared? Surprisingly, there are a lot of ways to enjoy this nutritious, leafy green veggie which includes;

- Spinach-artichoke dip,
- Creamed spinach,
- Spinach lasagna,
- Garlic sautéed spinach, and
- Spinach and cheese stuffed pasta shells.

Tea

Antioxidants in tea called *polyphenols and flavonoids* are known to boost the ability of the immune system.

Tea Time: A Cup of Immunity

About half of the population in America drinks tea regularly. *Antioxidants in tea called polyphenols and flavonoids are known to boost the ability of the immune system.*

These compounds can also reduce the risk of cardiovascular disease. Drinking green tea extract positively affects blood lipids, increasing good HDL cholesterol, and decreasing LDL bad cholesterol, triglycerides, and total cholesterol.

Beyond the Tea Cup

Tea is not only meant to be enjoyed from the cup. Amazingly, you should use teas in lots of your preferred recipes. Think beyond your cup!

- Put powdered tea to softened butter to produce a savory spread.
- Cook grains and noodles in tea rather than stock.
- Use powdered tea like a rub to infuse the meat with an unusual flavor.
- Help to make tea-infused dairy to use in cream sauces for pasta and rice dishes.
- Increase powdered tea to shortbread dough to make tea cookies.

Sweet Potatoes

Sweet potatoes have vitamins, and are cholesterol-free and fat-free food, providing helpful, immune-boosting benefits.

Say Yes to Sweet Potatoes

One medium sweet potato has an impressive 120% in the daily value of vitamin A and 30% in the daily value of vitamin C, all for 100 calories. These vitamins are necessary for immune function and ideal for your skin. Sweet potatoes are a cholesterol-free and fat-free food, and that means you get all of the helpful, immune-boosting vitamins with no guilt. Sweet potatoes contain healthy fiber too.

Sweet Potato Recipes to take Pleasure from

The deep, rich color of sweet potatoes reflects the high vitamin A content. These bright, orange root veggies can be whipped up in many ways. Try these nice potato dishes on for size.

- savory sweet potato fries.
- lovely potato casserole.
- twice baked special potatoes.
- sugary potato pie.

- great potato beet chips.

Broccoli

Broccoli is a nutrient-packed food with minerals and vitamins that help to maximize immune health.

Broccoli to the Rescue

Broccoli is a nutrient-packed food to aid your disease-fighting capability. One glass of broccoli provides just as much vitamin C as an orange. The veggie is saturated in beta-carotene, potassium, magnesium, zinc, and iron. Broccoli supplies a range of B vitamins (B1, B2, B3, and B6). Together, these minerals and vitamins help the disease-fighting capability to work to the best of its ability. Another healthy compound provided by broccoli: *glutathione*, the master antioxidant in the body.

Five Ways to Enjoy Broccoli

Not a fan of broccoli? Some people think it's great, some hate it, but broccoli is such a nutritious vegetable, it seems sensible to discover a way to eat even more of it. Broccoli can be prepared with techniques that are so tasty and will make you crave for it! You can try a broccoli dish in different ways:

- creamy broccoli and cheese soup.
- broccoli casserole.
- broccoli salad.
- lemon braised broccoli.
- roasted broccoli rabe.

Garlic

Antioxidant compounds in the ginger root have potent anti-inflammatory and immune-boosting properties.

Harness the Power of Garlic Cloves

Over the years, people have praised garlic due to its immune-boosting properties. Garlic has antibacterial, antiviral, and anti-fungal properties. The bulbs are abundant in antioxidants that quench free radicals that are likely involved in Alzheimer's disease, cardiovascular disease, cancers, and other situations. The antiviral properties can help to reduce the severity of colds, flu, or COVID-19 infections.

In a single study, people who took garlic supplements during the cold season caught fewer colds than those that took placebo pills. In case you are down with cold, garlic can help to shorten its duration. If you must try out garlic supplements, ensure the one you select contains the ingredients contained in the actual garlic.

Garlic and Cancer

Garlic improves the part of the disease-fighting ability that is tasked with fighting viruses and cancer. Several studies have documented a connection between the use of garlic and a reduced rate in different kinds of cancers. Individuals who eat lots of raw or cooked garlic regularly have 30% to 35% fewer colorectal cancers than those that do not take it at all. In a small study of people who had inoperable pancreatic, colorectal, or liver cancers, immune functioning was improved when participants took garlic extract for six months.

Miso soup

Miso soup is abundant with probiotics that are advantageous for gastrointestinal health and boosting the disease fighting capability.

Fermented Foods and Immunity

Miso soup has been a staple in Japanese cuisine for many years. *Miso is a salty paste made from fermented soybeans. It is abundant with probiotics that are advantageous for gastrointestinal health and boosting the disease fighting capability.*

A little bacteria or an imbalance of bacteria in the GI tract is associated with several medical ailments including irritable bowel syndrome (IBS), food allergies, gastroenteritis, inflammatory bowel disease (ulcerative colitis and Crohn's disease), as well as certain types of cancers. Drinking a cup of miso soup is a superb way to introduce beneficial food-based probiotics into the GI tract.

Busy Little Bugs

Beneficial micro-organisms in miso soup, and other fermented foods, perform several necessary functions in the GI tract. They synthesize vitamins and proteins. They produce short-chain essential fatty acids (SCFAs) that these cells are lining the GI tract use for fuel. The probiotics set up a healthy balance of flora in the gastrointestinal tract, avoiding pathogenic strains that make an effort to have held.

About 70% of the immune system is based on the gut. Healthy, balanced gut flora produces a strong disease-fighting capability.

Chicken Soup

Chicken soup decreases mucus and helps your body get rid of cold faster.

Serving a plate of relief

Scientists agree that chicken soup can help you overcome a cold faster. When cold viruses invade tissues from the upper respiratory system, your body responds by triggering inflammation. This inflammation signals white blood cells to go to the region and stimulates the production of mucus.

Ingredients in chicken soup can stop the movement of white blood cells, thereby decreasing mucus connected with colds.

Too tired to cook from the scratch?

Canned chicken soup can ease cold symptoms too.

More Cold-Fighting Remedies

To overcome cold quickly, *drink plenty of warm liquids like chicken soup, ginger tea, and tepid to warm water with lemon.* Staying hydrated helps thin mucus secretions and flushes the virus out of the body. Taking zinc lozenges, syrup, or tablets within a day of displaying cold symptoms might help decrease the duration of a cold. Taking vitamin C supplements throughout the cold might not prevent you from catching a cold.

However, it can help to ease the symptoms if you do catch one. It can also help to ease symptoms of flu and coronavirus infections.

Pomegranate

Pomegranate extracts possess antiviral properties to fight bad viruses and bacteria and promote the growth of effective gut flora.

Harness the Purple Power

Beneficial compounds in pomegranate extract have been used in lab studies to inhibit the growth of harmful types of bacteria, including Salmonella, Yersinia, Shigella, Listeria, Clostridium, Staphylococcus aureus, and other organisms. Also, there is evidence pomegranate compounds inhibit the growth of bacteria in the mouth that contribute to periodontal disease, plaque buildup, and gingivitis. Pomegranate extracts have antiviral properties contrary to flu, herpes, and other viruses.

Furthermore, to fight bad viruses and bacteria, there is evidence that pomegranate extracts promote the growth of beneficial gut flora that improves the disease-fighting capability, including *Bifidobacterium and Lactobacillus*.

Five ways to enjoy Pomegranate

A lot of people enjoy pomegranate by eating the jewel-colored seeds after cutting the fruit open. However, there are many other ways to enjoy pomegranate.

- Add more tart, colorful pomegranate seeds to the fruit salad.
- Cool off with pomegranate lemonade on hot summer days.
- Make a nice salad with watercress, endive, blood oranges, and pomegranate seeds.
- Mix pomegranate seeds into wild rice pilaf.
- Use pomegranate seeds to prepare a tasty relish to top meats.

Ginger

Antioxidant compounds in ginger root have potent anti-inflammatory and immune-boosting properties.

Anti-inflammatory Root

Antioxidant compounds in the ginger root have potent anti-inflammatory and immune-boosting properties. Normal metabolic processes in the body, infections, and toxins all contribute to the production of free radicals leading to oxidative stress. Antioxidants in foods like ginger reduce free radicals and help to protect the body from arthritis, cancer, neurodegenerative disorders, and many other conditions.

Grate some fresh ginger and steep it in hot water to make tea. Freshly grated ginger also makes a great addition to healthy stir-fried veggies. Ginger has proven antibacterial and antiviral properties.

Five ways to eat Ginger

What can you do with ginger root?

A whole lot! Here are some ideas to help you add more ginger to your menu.

- Add ginger to hot chocolate for a quick shot.
- Grated ginger makes a good combination with carrot cake or spice muffins.
- Make a ginger orange glaze to take pleasure from over salmon filets.
- Mix ginger with marinades for meat.
- Enjoy honey ginger chicken wings.

Maximizing the fitness of your immune system is simple

when you understand which foods to eat.

Eat these 16 immune-boosting foods to keep your disease fighting capability working effectively.

Other Foods that Boost and Increase Your Immune System

Elderberry

Extracts of elderberry have antiviral, anticancer, and anti-inflammatory properties.

Elderberry is a plant that is being used medicinally for many years. Sambucus nigra, or black elderberry bush, is the variety that is mostly used to create syrup and lozenges. Extracts of elderberry have antiviral, anticancer, and anti-inflammatory properties.

Elderberry is saturated with flavonoids. People take elderberry syrup as a cure for colds, flu, and bacterial sinus infections.

The medicinal plant functions by reducing swelling in the mucus membranes. Some studies suggest that the juice gotten from elderberry reduces the duration of the flu. If it works for flu infections, it can help your immune system to fight against coronavirus (COVID-19) infection.

Elderberry Interactions

Elderberry has numerous benefits; however, the cure may only work together with some specifically prescribed drugs. Always check with your doctor or pharmacist before adding a new drug or cure to your routine.

Elderberry may not work with the following medications.

Diuretics: Elderberry is a diuretic, so taking it with a drug that has a diuretic prescription, increases the effects.

Laxatives: Elderberry has laxative effects so it shouldn't be taken with other laxative mediations.

Steroids: Elderberry stimulates the immune system, so it shouldn't be taken with steroids alongside other medications made to suppress the disease-fighting capability of the body. People who are on immunosuppressive drugs after having undergone organ transplant shouldn't consider elderberry.

Chemotherapy: Elderberry may hinder chemotherapy and should not be used with it.

Diabetes medications: Elderberry lowers blood sugar levels, so it shouldn't be taken with drugs that treat diabetes.

Theophylline: Elderberry may reduce blood degrees of this drug required to take care of asthma and respiratory conditions.

Mushrooms

Mushrooms are rich in selenium and B vitamins like riboflavin and niacin, which are necessary for the immune defense to be able to work effectively.

Wondering how you can boost your immune system? Eat more button mushrooms. Mushrooms are also rich in polysaccharides, sugar-like substances that boost immune function.

Flavorful Fungus

Mushrooms have a savory quality that can improve the flavor of several dishes. Not sure of how to eat mushrooms? Try the following mouth-watering steps to have these tasty fungi:

Sautéing, barbecuing, and roasting can help to draw out the rich, savory flavor of mushrooms.

Mushrooms make an excellent addition to scrambled eggs and omelets.

Toss sliced mushrooms into soups, salads, or lasagna.

Enjoy Portobello mushroom tops in veggie burgers.

Stuffed mushrooms make tasty hors d'oeuvres.

Acai Berry

The acai berry is rich in anthocyanins that are flavonoid substances that combat oxidative stress in the body and reduce inflammation.

Acai Berry Pulp Benefits

Acai berry is a black-purple fruit that is gotten from the acai berry palm tree in Brazil, Trinidad, and some parts of South USA. The fruit is rich in anthocyanins. These flavonoid substances are very powerful antioxidants. They combat oxidative stress in the body by mopping up free radicals. Antioxidants are known for boosting immunity and reducing inflammation in the body. There is never a better time to take pleasure from an acai bowl than now!

Immune-Boosting Fruit

Acai berry pulp is a potent antioxidant and stimulator of the immune system, and researchers are examining it as a potential treatment for all sorts of conditions. Parts of the report include the use of acai in people with:

- ❖ increasing prostate-specific antigen (PSA);
- ❖ Coronary disease and metabolic syndrome;
- ❖ Lower rectum cancer;

❖ Constipation, and

Another prospect of studies could include other conditions (for instance, yeast-based infections, Flu, COVID-19).

Oysters

Oysters provide selenium, iron, vitamin C and A, zinc, and high-quality protein for proper immune function.

Oysters are a nutritional powerhouse from the ocean. One 3-ounce serving of Pacific oysters provides 190% in the daily value of selenium, 45% of the daily value of iron, and 20% on the daily value of vitamin C, all for 140 calories. One 3-ounce serving of oysters contains 16 grams of high-quality protein. The seafood also contains zinc and vitamin A. These minerals and vitamins in oysters are crucial for proper immune function.

Ways to eat Oysters

Many people are familiar with raw oysters served with the half shell, but you will discover that there are several other methods of eating oysters. They include;

- Oysters Rockefeller,
- Oyster Stew,
- Oyster Stuffing,
- Scalloped Oysters, And
- Grilled Oysters.

Watermelon

Watermelon provides the body with vitamins A, C, and B6, nutrients, and compounds like glutathione for proper immune functioning.

Pumped About Watermelon

Watermelon Nutrition

Watermelon is an immune-boosting fruit. One 2-cup serving of watermelon has 270 mg of potassium, 30% from the daily value of vitamin A, and 25% of the worth of vitamin C. Calories in watermelon aren't much. One 2-cup serving of watermelon has just 80 calories. Watermelon also provides vitamin B6 and glutathione. Your body needs these vitamins, nutrients, and compounds like glutathione for proper immune function.

Five ways to eat Watermelon

Watermelon slices is the most typical way to take pleasure from this fruit. Here are some creative ways to eat watermelon.

Make a fruit salad with watermelon and top it with lemon, honey, and mint dressing.
Take a tall glass of watermelon strawberry lemonade.
Snack on arugula watermelon salad topped with feta cheese.
Enjoy frozen watermelon sorbet.
Cool-down with watermelon, ginger, lime pops.

Wheat Germ

Wheat germ is rich in B vitamins, zinc, and vitamin E and helps boost nutrition when added to foods.

Wheat germ is the innermost part of the wheat kernel and it is the most nutritious part of the grain. The germ is rich in B vitamins, zinc, and vitamin E. Sprinkle wheat germ with yogurt or cereal and bring it to some shake.

Wheat germ is a good way to boost the nourishment of cooked goods. Substitute wheat germ for any bit of bleached flour in recipes to get some good extra minerals and vitamins.

What now with Wheat Germ?

A lot of people know that wheat germ makes a very tasty topping when sprinkled on fruit, yogurt, or cereal, but what else can be done with it? Wheat germ is a versatile food that can be used in several recipes.

Combine wheat germ, herbs, and spices to make a breaded coating for baked chicken and fish.

Use wheat germ instead of breadcrumbs in meatloaf and meatballs.

Sprinkle wheat germ with baked apple crumble and similar desserts.

Yogurt

Yogurt is rich in probiotics and vitamins that can greatly help to boost immunity.

Reasons to like Low-Fat Yogurt

Nourishment guidelines recommend that adults consume three servings of milk products each day. Low-fat yogurt provides 11 grams of protein, 250 calories, and almost 400 mg of calcium per 8-ounce serving. Low-fat yogurt may also help to meet your daily requirement of vitamin B12, vitamin D, and vitamin B2 (riboflavin). Adequate quantities of vitamin D, as well as other nutrients, are essential for robust immune function.

Yogurt is rich in probiotics, including Lactobacillus acidophilus, Lactobacillus casei, and Bifidus. These strains boost immune function and can even lessen both the length and severity of colds. Beneficial gut flora is necessary for proper digestion, detoxification, and immune function. Probiotics even lessen eczema symptoms in babies.

Five ways to eat Yogurt

A lot of people eat yogurt straight from the cup, but you can find many other methods to enjoy this immune-boosting food.

Mix yogurt, juice, and a little bit of honey together. Pour into molds and freeze to create yogurt pops.
Enjoy cucumber salad with yogurt dill dressing.
Get coleslaw with yogurt rather than mayonnaise.
Serve fish topped with minted yogurt sauce.
Use yogurt in creamy soup recipes to give them a tart kick.

Spinach

Spinach contains folate, vitamin A, vitamin C, fiber, magnesium, and iron to improve immune functioning.
Super Spinach
Leafy Green Superfood

Spinach is rated as a superfood due to the high level of folate, vitamin A, vitamin C, fiber, magnesium, and iron it contains. The nutrients in spinach boost the immune system and provide your body with the necessary nutrients for cell division and DNA repair. Get maximum advantages from spinach by eating it raw or slightly cooked to preserve nutrients.

Think beyond Spinach Salad

Many people are familiar with spinach salad, but how else can spinach be prepared? Surprisingly, there are a lot of ways to enjoy this nutritious, leafy green veggie which includes;

- Spinach-artichoke dip,
- Creamed spinach,
- Spinach lasagna,
- Garlic sautéed spinach, and
- Spinach and cheese stuffed pasta shells.

Tea

Antioxidants in tea called polyphenols and flavonoids are known to boost the ability of the immune system.

Tea Time: A Cup of Immunity

About half of the population in America drinks tea regularly. Antioxidants in tea called polyphenols and flavonoids are known to boost the ability of the immune system.

These compounds can also reduce the risk of cardiovascular disease. Drinking green tea extract positively affects blood lipids, increasing good HDL cholesterol, and decreasing LDL bad cholesterol, triglycerides, and total cholesterol.

Beyond the Tea Cup

Tea is not only meant to be enjoyed from the cup. Amazingly, you should use teas in lots of your preferred recipes. Think beyond your cup!

- Put powdered tea to softened butter to produce a savory spread.
- Cook grains and noodles in tea rather than stock.
- Use powdered tea like a rub to infuse the meat with an unusual flavor.
- Help to make tea-infused dairy to use in cream sauces for pasta and rice dishes.
- Increase powdered tea to shortbread dough to make tea cookies.

Sweet Potatoes

Sweet potatoes have vitamins, and are cholesterol-free and fat-free food, providing helpful, immune-boosting benefits.

Say Yes to Sweet Potatoes

One medium sweet potato has an impressive 120% in the daily value of vitamin A and 30% in the daily value of vitamin C, all for 100 calories. These vitamins are necessary for immune function and ideal for your skin. Sweet potatoes are a cholesterol-free and fat-free food, and that means you get all of the helpful, immune-boosting vitamins with no guilt. Sweet potatoes contain healthy fiber too.

Sweet potato recipes to take pleasure from

The deep, rich color of sweet potatoes reflects the high vitamin A content. These bright, orange root veggies can be whipped up in many ways. Try these nice potato dishes on for size.

- savory sweet potato fries
- lovely potato casserole
- twice baked special potatoes
- sugary potato pie
- great potato beet chips

Broccoli

Broccoli is a nutrient-packed food with minerals and vitamins that help to maximize immune health.

Broccoli to the Rescue

Broccoli is a nutrient-packed food to aid your disease-fighting capability. One glass of broccoli provides just as much vitamin C as an orange. The veggie is saturated in beta-carotene, potassium, magnesium, zinc, and iron. Broccoli supplies a range of B vitamins (B1, B2, B3, and B6). Together, these minerals and vitamins help the disease-fighting capability to work to the best of its ability. Another healthy compound provided by broccoli: glutathione, the master antioxidant in the body.

Five ways to enjoy Broccoli

Not a fan of broccoli? Some people think it's great, some hate it, but broccoli is such a nutritious vegetable, it seems sensible to discover a way to eat even more of it. Broccoli can be prepared with techniques that are so tasty and will make you crave for it! You can try a broccoli dish in different ways:

- creamy broccoli and cheese soup

- broccoli casserole
- broccoli salad
- lemon braised broccoli
- roasted broccoli rabe

Garlic

Antioxidant compounds in the ginger root have potent anti-inflammatory and immune-boosting properties.

Harness the energy of Garlic Cloves

Over the years, people have praised garlic due to its immune-boosting properties. Garlic has antibacterial, antiviral, and anti-fungal properties. The bulbs are abundant in antioxidants that quench free radicals that are likely involved in Alzheimer's disease, cardiovascular disease, cancers, and other situations. The antiviral properties can help to reduce the severity of colds, flu, or COVID-19 infections.

In a single study, people who took garlic supplements during the cold season caught fewer colds than those that took placebo pills. In case you are down with cold, garlic can help to shorten its duration. If you must try out garlic supplements, ensure the one you select contains the ingredients contained in the actual garlic.

Garlic and Cancer

Garlic improves the part of the disease-fighting ability that is tasked with fighting viruses and cancer. Several studies have documented a connection between the use of garlic and a reduced rate in different kinds of cancers. Individuals who eat lots of raw or cooked garlic regularly have 30% to 35% fewer colorectal cancers than those that do not take it at all. In a small study of people who had inoperable pancreatic, colorectal, or liver cancers, immune functioning was improved when participants took garlic extract for six months.

Miso soup

Miso soup is abundant with probiotics that are advantageous for gastrointestinal health and boosting the disease fighting capability.

Fermented Foods and Immunity

Miso soup has been a staple in Japanese cuisine for many years. Miso is a salty paste made from fermented soybeans. It is abundant with probiotics that are advantageous for gastrointestinal health and boosting the disease fighting capability.

A little bacteria or an imbalance of bacteria in the GI tract is associated with several medical ailments including irritable bowel syndrome (IBS), food allergies, gastroenteritis, inflammatory bowel disease (ulcerative colitis and Crohn's disease), as well as certain types of cancers. Drinking a cup of miso soup is a superb way to introduce beneficial food-based probiotics into the GI tract.

Busy Little Bugs

Beneficial microorganisms in miso soup, and other fermented foods, perform several necessary functions in the GI tract. They synthesize vitamins and proteins. They produce short-chain essential fatty acids (SCFAs) that these cells are lining the GI tract use for fuel. The probiotics set up a healthy balance of flora in the gastrointestinal tract, avoiding pathogenic strains that make an effort to have held. About 70% of the immune system is based on the gut. Healthy, balanced gut flora produces a strong disease-fighting capability.

Chicken soup

Chicken soup decreases mucus and helps your body get rid of cold faster.

Serving a plate of relief

Scientists agree that chicken soup can help you overcome a cold faster. When cold viruses invade tissues from the upper respiratory system, your body responds by triggering inflammation. This inflammation signals white blood cells to go to the region and stimulates the production of mucus. Ingredients in chicken soup can stop the movement of white blood cells, thereby decreasing mucus connected with colds.

Too tired to cook from the scratch? Canned chicken soup can ease cold symptoms too.

More Cold-Fighting Remedies

To overcome cold quickly, drink plenty of warm liquids like chicken soup, ginger tea, and tepid to warm water with lemon. Staying hydrated helps thin mucus secretions and flushes the virus out of the body. Taking zinc lozenges, syrup, or tablets within a day of displaying cold symptoms might help decrease the duration of a cold. Taking vitamin C supplements throughout the cold might not prevent you from catching a cold.

However, it can help to ease the symptoms if you do catch one. It can also help to ease symptoms of flu and coronavirus infections.

Pomegranate

Pomegranate extracts possess antiviral properties to fight bad viruses and bacteria and promote the growth of effective gut flora.

Harness the Purple Power

Beneficial compounds in pomegranate extract have been used in lab studies to inhibit the growth of harmful types of bacteria, including E Coli O157:H7, Salmonella, Yersinia, Shigella, Listeria, Clostridium, Staphylococcus aureus, and other organisms. Also, there is evidence pomegranate compounds inhibit the growth of bacteria in the mouth that contribute to periodontal disease, plaque buildup, and gingivitis. Pomegranate extracts have antiviral properties contrary to flu, herpes, and other viruses. Furthermore, to fight bad viruses and bacteria, there is evidence that pomegranate extracts promote the growth of beneficial gut flora that improves the disease-fighting capability, including Bifidobacterium and Lactobacillus.

Five ways to enjoy Pomegranate

A lot of people enjoy pomegranate by eating the jewel-colored seeds after cutting the fruit open. However, there are many other ways to enjoy pomegranate.

- Add more tart, colorful pomegranate seeds to the fruit salad.
- Cool off with pomegranate lemonade on hot summer days.
- Make a nice salad with watercress, endive, blood oranges, and pomegranate seeds.
- Mix pomegranate seeds into wild rice pilaf.
- Use pomegranate seeds to prepare a tasty relish to top meats.

Ginger

Antioxidant compounds in ginger root have potent anti-inflammatory and immune-boosting properties.

Anti-inflammatory Root

Antioxidant compounds in the ginger root have potent anti-inflammatory and immune-boosting properties. Normal metabolic processes in the body, infections, and toxins all contribute to the production of free radicals leading to oxidative stress. Antioxidants in foods like ginger reduce free radicals and help to protect the body from arthritis, cancer, neurodegenerative disorders, and many other conditions.

Grate some fresh ginger and steep it in hot water to make tea. Freshly grated ginger also makes a great addition to healthy stir-fried veggies. Ginger has proven antibacterial and antiviral properties.

Five ways to eat Ginger

What can you do with ginger root? A whole lot! Here are some ideas to help you add more ginger to your menu.

- Add ginger to hot chocolate for a quick shot.
- Grated ginger makes a good combination with carrot cake or spice muffins.
- Make a ginger orange glaze to take pleasure from over salmon filets.
- Mix ginger with marinades for meat.

- Enjoy honey ginger chicken wings.

Maximizing the fitness of your immune system is simple when you understand which foods to eat.

Eat these 16 immune-boosting foods to keep your disease fighting capability working effectively.

Chapter 4
Immune Boosting Foods, Tonics & Teas.

It's that time of year again; the sniffles are starting, the coughs continuing, plus never-ending nausea. Cold and flu season is upon us. Whether you are vulnerable to falling sick or can steer clear of the illnesses most of the year, it is still essential to prevent cold and flu.

Not only can cold or flu be a nuisance, by interrupting your lifestyle and routines, and causing you to feel awful, but it is also a symptom of a weak immune system.

A weak immune system can also be associated with high degrees of stress, poor sleep, and poor digestion. So, addressing many of these things might help to strengthen your disease-fighting capability amazingly. However, there are foods, herbs, tonics, and teas that you can use to strengthen your disease-fighting capability to prevent you from falling sick, and besides, there are also foods you can eat to recuperate if you are already sick. From fruits and vegetables to extracts and tinctures, continue reading for list of most effective immune-boosting foods, including tonics, teas, and many more!

Fruits

Just like vegetables, fruits are more beneficial to our health, wellness, and immune system when they are grown organically. Especially fruits like berries, which are generally on the dirty dozen list yet so saturated in things such as antioxidants, vitamins, and nutrients. Choose your fruits organically to avoid the effects of pesticides and chemicals, which increase the toxic load and can burden the immune system. And, just like vegetables, certain fruits have amazing immune-boosting benefits that you might not know about. Read on and enjoy these powerful items for maximum immunity!

Coconuts & Coconut Oil

Coconuts and Coconut Oil:

Coconut in every of its forms is a super-food powerhouse. It is filled with healthy essential fatty acids, that is effective for metabolism, and can be used as a beauty product for healthier hair and skin, and today you can add *"immune-boosting"* to the list of benefits.

Coconut oil has been proven to contain antimicrobial that kills fungus and bacteria and has proven useful in helping to fight pneumonia. One study showed that children who took coconut oil recovered from pneumonia faster than those that didn't and also had reduced fevers, clearer breathing, and normal blood oxygenation. The next time you add coconut oil to your smoothie or cooked veggies, your immune system will thank you!

Berries

Berries:

Berries, such as blueberries, raspberries, strawberries, and blackberries, are on top of the ORAC scale - meaning they contain a few of the highest amounts of antioxidants that help to fight free radicals. This is ideal for your defense mechanisms and health and wellness. Blueberries, in particular, can help you resist colds and flu, though, as they are high in pterostilbene. Researchers from Oregon State University found that when this compound was combined with vitamin D, the body's ability to resist illness increased. The same was shown with the resveratrol found in red grapes. Yet another reason to enjoy those blueberries!

Citrus Fruits

Citric Fruits:

Citric fruits, like grapefruit, oranges, and lemons, are low in sugar, which may be immune-suppressant, and filled with vitamin C, which is vital for defending the body against infections like colds and flu by increasing the production of white blood cells. The body cannot produce vitamin C on its own, so ensure you get enough vitamin C by taking fruits and vegetables like citrus fruits which are filled with this immune-boosting vitamin!

Apples

Apples:

Aside from being filled with vitamin C, apples are also a rich way to obtain soluble fiber. A report in 2010 carried out by the University of Illinois showed that dietary fiber helps to fortify the immune system by changing the "personalities" of immune cells. Rather than being pro-inflammatory, the cells consider anti-inflammatory, healing cells that help your body to get over infection and illness faster. I guess the old saying is a right "an apple a day keeps the doctor away!"

Teas

What is better than curling up on a couch with a mug of tea when you are down with a cold or flu? You definitely do this for reasons beyond taking comfort.

Teas are a good way to transform your disease-fighting capability and battle common cold symptoms. They have different properties that can help to cure things like sore throat, stomach upset, and congestion. Also, many teas help you to relax and drift off into sleep, which is one of their most important benefits.

Stock your cupboards and revel in these in sickness and in health!

Ginger Tea

You can make your ginger tea by grating fresh ginger and steeping it in warm water with some lemon. This produces a delicious tea that is soothing for the throat and is also ideal for helping nausea or digestive issues. You can even buy a selection of ginger teas that have the same anti-microbial and anti-viral effects as the main element.

Holy Basil (*Tulsi Tea*)

This is a multi-purpose tea that will help with a lot of things. One of the uses of holy basil tea is to help with respiratory disorders when you are sick.

Although it is also good for fever, asthma, lung disorders, cardiovascular disease, and stress. Holy basil is another amazing herb that can help to relieve stress and support your adrenal glands, which indirectly helps to support the immune system.

Brew a cup and sip it slowly then you'll understand why it is referred to as being calming and soothing.

Mint

Mint is probably one of the most popular teas. Not only does it taste great and help you to keep your breath fresh, but its strong aroma and flavor can also help to soothe sore throats and heal anyone faster from respiratory ailments. And, it can help you feel revitalized and refreshed, so if you're battling with cold, a warm mug of mint tea will give you the boost you need to conquer it forever.

Chamomile

Chamomile tea is usually used as a night-time tea when people need to relax or need help with sleeping.

It is ideal for its relaxing and mood-soothing benefits, as is the gas of chamomile in a diffuser. However, chamomile tea can be helpful to calm stomach upset, which explains why many people use it when they have colds or flu. It's an all-natural tea that, like ginger, that can calm or soothe nausea or indigestion.

Lavender

One of the most remarkable features of lavender is stress. It can help to alleviate stress and increase relaxation, which is necessary when you're under the weather. It is also ideal for helping to promote peaceful rest, which can seem evasive when you have a cold or flu. Most people like soaking Epsom salts and some lavender oil in the bath when they're sick and lavender tea is another smart way to derive pleasure from its benefits. Plus, it's been proven to greatly help to soothe stomach bloating!

Use these different foods, herbs, and ideas to strengthen your immune system this season and prevent catching that pesky cold or nasty flu. <u>And understand that the main</u>

element of laying a healthy foundation for the immune system is a healthy diet plan, reduced stress, and adequate sleep.

Vegetables

First on our list is vegetables. Where else would we start? Vegetables have a lot of amazing ability to impact and improve our health and wellness. We have four as our favorites for immune-boosting benefits, however before we proceed, let's discuss the need for organic.

Certified organic produce is the best option you can make for your health. It helps to ensure that you get the nutrients you need from organic soil, whereas conventional produce is grown on mineral-depleted and nutrient-starved soils. Certified organic produce is grown and farmed without the use of chemicals or pesticides.

Actually, by choosing the Dirty Dozen (the 12 most dirty vegetables & fruits) organic, you could reduce your pesticide intake by 80%. Vegetables have a lot to offer, particularly when it involves immune benefits, but make sure you're taking advantage of your veggies by choosing organic!

Cabbage

Cabbage is a cruciferous vegetable that comes in many colors and is low in calories but highly filled with nutrients, including vitamin C which has about 37mg per 100g of cabbage. And vitamin C is a crucial nutrient with regards to immunity!

When raw, it is very healthy, cabbage is best for the immune system and digestive tract when it's fermented in the form of sauerkraut or kimchi. Fermented foods heal the gut lining and aid digestion, and your gut properties 70% of your immune system cells, meaning fermented foods boost your immunity too.

Garlic

Garlic:

You might have heard about using garlic to defend yourself against deficiencies, but have you thought about using them to protect yourself against colds and flu?

Garlic contains compounds that have been proven to improve white blood cells' ability to fight off some viruses, especially the ones responsible for colds and flu. It's great to eat, but it also comes in supplement form, and studies show that daily supplementation with garlic can reduce colds by 63% in comparison to placebo; another study showed that a high dose of garlic extract can reduce the number of cold or flu days by 61%. It's a powerhouse for your immune system!

Red Pepper

Peppers:

Another vegetable that is full of immune-boosting vitamin C is bell peppers. Red bell peppers are richer in vitamin C than most of the other varieties, bell peppers also provide lots of phytochemicals and carotenoids, like beta-carotene, that are filled with antioxidants and anti-inflammatory benefits too. Also, peppers can help to clear out congested mucus **membranes** in the nose and lungs, helping you to eliminate the toxins and disease-causing components of your cold or flu faster!

Spinach

Spinach:

Similar to cabbage and peppers, spinach is also filled with vitamin C, which helps to fight cold and flu and strengthen the disease-fighting capability. That's not all; it is also saturated in antioxidants and beta-carotene, like peppers, which can help our disease-fighting capability fight infection and viruses easier. A fascinating fact about spinach is that its nutrients are best retained when the vegetable is raw, so try to enjoy spinach in a delicious salad instead of stir fry to get the most immune benefits out of it.

Avoid milk and sugar at the first sign of any cold sickness. Milk thickens fluids in you, allowing the mucus to stick in the ears, nose, throat, and chest- an ideal place for nasty bugs to grow and multiply.

Refined, processed sugar (only less than a teaspoon) weakens your disease-fighting capability and serves as food for the unwanted microbes.

Tinctures & Extracts

Just like herbs, *tinctures, and extracts* are a powerful way to boost health but they usually contain more potency. Tinctures and extracts provide a unique way for your body to soak up compounds that may not be easily available through drinking extraction and raise the potency and benefits of these compounds compared to when they are not in tincture or extract form. Besides, tinctures and extracts are available in single distillations, such as only astragalus, or mixtures, like in Deep Immune, to help harness the energy of different multiple compounds into one amazing product. Ask us about tinctures and extracts so we can help you find the appropriate one for you!

Astragalus

Astragalus can be an adaptogen, meaning it can help your body balance what needs balancing: lowering what is high and increasing what is low. Adaptogens protect your body against various stresses, including physical, mental, and emotional - and yes, the immune system is usually also protected. It is known to prevent colds and upper respiratory infections, and contain antiviral homes that support, and stimulate the disease fighting capability. You'll find astragalus in almost every type of extract and tinctures, but Deep Immune by St. Francis is a great combination that has astragalus and helps to strengthen a weak immune system. It's ideal for this time of the year!

Oregano Oil

Oregano oil is categorized as the heavy hitter for colds and flu. Made from the leaves and flowers of Oregano, which you can use in your cooking, oregano oil comes in tincture and extracts variety to aid in boosting your immune system. One research conducted in the George Town University Infirmary showed that oregano oil can overcome harmful organism infections, making it capable of defending the body against things like salmonella and E. coli. It is perhaps one of the most effective remedies that is used to improve the body's natural immunity and that can also be used in many ways, including inhalation.

Mushroom Extracts

Mushrooms contain a few of the most powerful natural medicines on earth, and one of their benefits is their capability to boost the immune system. Immune 7 by Purica contains the energy of 6 different medicinal mushrooms to provide full-spectrum immune support. In addition to these powerful mushrooms, Immune 7 also includes Nutricol, which is Purica's mixture of super-strength antioxidants. Together, these ingredients give a powerhouse supplement to improve and increase your immunity!

Echinacea extract

Echinacea is a healthy extract that helps with lung support and bronchial infections. It is typically known to shorten the duration of the normal cold and flu, as well as reduce symptoms like sore throat, cough, and fever. Anti-Viral by Natural Factors is a potent tincture that richly contains *Echinaceato* to support and fight colds.

Herbs

I understand how much energy is needed to maintain our general health and improve it when things are going awry. People often turns to herbs, using spices and teas to help her cope with different health problems, and encourages others to do the same. Herbs are especially important when it comes to our immune system and they are always within our reach! Using them to cook whether in dried or fresh forms or using them in oils and tinctures, you can't go wrong if you choose to add more herbs to your everyday life. Continue reading for top immune-boosting herbs and start using them in your kitchen.

Oregano

Oregano:

Herbs are powerful with regards to our health and wellness, and oregano is a superb one for immune benefits. It's saturated in vitamins A, C, E, and K, which are best for the immune system, and features anti-inflammatory, anti-microbial, and anti-fungal effects. Studies show that essential oils from oregano can help to fight off Listeria and the superbug MRSA. Imagine what it can do for your everyday immune health!

Turmeric

Turmeric:

You've probably heard of turmeric as a superfood herb, with its high antioxidant and anti-inflammatory properties. But do you know the active component that helps with this stuff in turmeric is called *curcumin*?

This is an anti-viral, anti-fungal, anti-inflammatory compound that is excellent in resisting everyday colds and flu as well as more serious conditions like cancer. Plus, since inflammation is the cause of so many diseases, being anti-inflammatory is a bonus.

Ginger

Ginger:

Ginger is historically one of the most common substances used to help against colds and flu. It is a healthy agent to assist, defend against, and dispel nausea because of its ability to support break up and dispelling ff intestinal gas or other disruptions. It is a good remedy to have when you are down with flu, as in lemon and ginger tea, or for chewing the way people chew it. Also, because it is good for nausea, it is known to be effective for traveling sickness, seasickness, and sickness associated with pregnancy.

Licorice Root

Licorice root:

Licorice is good for a lot of ailments, and one amazing power they have is to improve the adrenals and support the strain response. Your adrenal system is intricately associated with your disease-fighting capability. When you're too stressed and your adrenals are worn out, your defense mechanisms are more susceptible to attack. Helping to strengthen your adrenals and stress response is a good way to support your immune system! Plus, licorice has been known to enhance immunity more directly by boosting immune system chemicals that help to flush out viruses.

Chapter 5
Bitters for Immune Health

Drink bitters for an immune boost. This healthy tonic is made from *astragalus root, ginger, angelica root, and honey* - all ingredients which can help the immune system to keep working efficiently.

Astragalus, a prominent herb in Chinese medicine, contains anti-inflammatory and antibacterial properties. Studies on astragalus claim that the root can enhance resistance to infections and regulate the body's immune responses.

Also, ***Angelica roots*** have been proven to regulate the immune system and treat respiratory ailments and cold symptoms.

Lastly, both ***Ginger and Honey*** are powerful antioxidants that contain anti-inflammatory and antibacterial properties.

Honey activates the immune system's response to infection and prevents cell proliferation. Similarly, *ginger* also provides anti-inflammatory effects and can help with muscle pain.

Recipe for Immune-Boosting Bitters

Ingredients:

1 tbsp. honey

1 oz. dried astragalus root

1 oz. dried angelica root

1/2 oz. dried chamomile

1 tsp. dried ginger

1 tsp. dried orange peel

One cinnamon stick

1 tsp. cardamom seeds

10 oz. alcohol (recommended: 100 proof vodka)

Steps:

- Melt the honey in 2 teaspoons of boiling water. Allow it to cool.
- Mix the honey and seven other ingredients in a mason jar and pour alcohol on top.
- Seal tightly and store the bitters in a cool, dark place.
- Allow bitters to infuse for about 2-4 weeks so the potency can be achieved. Shake the jars regularly (about once daily).

- When ready, sieve the bitters with a muslin cheesecloth or coffee filter. Store the sieved bitters in an airtight container at room temperature.

To Use:

Mix this tonic into hot tea or take a few drops as soon as you get out of bed for protection during cold and flu season.

Q: Any kind of concerns or health reasons someone shouldn't be taking these bitters?

A: Bitters should be avoided by pregnant women and nursing mothers. This recipe specifically contains dried angelica root which can stimulate uterine contractions and increase the threat of miscarriage. When the angelic root is consumed, your skin might be very sensitive to sunlight; therefore, daily sunscreen is recommended.

Herbs

It's that season of the year to use the boots, light the fireplace, and restock your over-the-counter cold medicine.

But maybe this season you're not thinking about the de rigueur drowsiness that comes with Tylenol Cold or the sugary aftertaste of Emergen-C. If so, consider the use of plants to boost your immunity and help you hedge infections.

Yep, this is one way to make a cold/flu season medical kit with herbs.

Solutions made from herbs and plants are a modality filled with powerful allies for your wellbeing and immunity, explains Sarah Corbett, Atlanta-based clinical herbalist at Rowan and Sage - and science is beginning to agree: *"Research is starting to confirm the efficacy of medicines people have been using for more than 100 years,"* says Corbett.

Listed below are six easy herbal supplements you can add to your medicine cabinet (or fridge, as it might be).

Get the Energy Combo

Herbs can supply your immune system with a little boost. Every year the flu shot is updated to better fight viruses in the body, because yes, the virus gets stronger, and so should you. Get the flu shot.

1. Elderberry

It's likely you have already tried elderberry in a few types or another, as this deep-purple berry has gained prominence over the last couple of years.

Also known as Sambucus, elderberry is antifungal, antibacterial, and antimicrobial, so it is efficient at knocking out almost every disease in the body. There is also evidence that elderberry works well in treating flu.
It is mostly found in syrup (it'll help to make your kitchen smell pleasant if you DIY), but tinctures (a plant extract made out of alcohol or glycerin), lozenges, and gummies can work too.

Take this remedy once daily if you're trying to avoid sickness, and more frequently (like every few hours) when you are sick.

Elderberry is known to be safe, but don't chug a whole bottle or anything close to it. One teaspoon or two or more tablespoons of syrup at the same time will work. Store syrups in the fridge because they are not shelf-reliant. When you have any autoimmune disorders, it is probably better to avoid them (since it stimulates the disease-fighting capability).

2. Echinacea

Another popular immune booster is echinacea, aka coneflower. It works by revitalizing the immune system to produce natural killer cells and other disease-fighters.

A 2015 meta-analysis figured echinacea might benefit people with low immune function the most, actually reducing the chance to get cold for as much as 35 percent.

It is best to use *echinacea* the moment you begin to feel something tickling in your throat rather than wait till when it is fully-blown.

A tincture is the best way to think of it, but teas won't fail you either (since you'll be hydrating your body most of the time). Look for **Echinacea Angustifolia** or a complete plant extract, because it's one of the most chemically bioavailable (very easily absorbed and used by the body).

Note that when you have an allergy to ragweed, you might be sensitive to *echinacea*, <u>if you notice any allergic reactions like itchiness, hives, or increased congestion, discontinue it immediately.</u>

When you have an autoimmune disorder, don't take echinacea.

3. Ginger

Yes, ginger will soothe an upset stomach, but it is also ideal for boosting your immunity during cold and flu season.

This versatile plant (which is known to be antimicrobial, antibiotic, and anti-inflammatory) lends its natural fire to different uses, sip the ginger tea, check out the juice bar for a new ginger shot if you're feeling icky, or simply use more ginger in your cooking.

It's fairly safe when used in cooking and solutions, but pregnant people shouldn't take more than 2 grams of dried ginger daily.

4. Garlic

Garlic's powers go beyond making food taste delicious. It's thought to stimulate the disease-fighting capability and raise the efficacy of white blood cells, though studies are inconclusive.

Garlic is simple to use - eat it daily to remain at the top of your health game. Also; up your garlic intake when you're sick. Use it to make a brilliant garlicky soup (don't skimp on the bone broth, either), eat several raw garlic cloves, roast a garlic bulb, or pack it into a jar of honey and allow it to sit for a couple of weeks to infuse.

Dietary doses of garlic are pretty safe. It might be difficult to take enough to harm you, but if you're on anti-clotting medications, be careful. (And remember to brush your teeth when you are going on top of the hog with raw garlic).

5. Fire cider

This intense liquid, sometimes also known as the Master Tonic, is kitchen medicine at its best: a precise combination of garlic, ginger, onion, horseradish, and chilly peppers (plus a variety of other immune-boosting ingredients like turmeric, or tasty ones like lemon or rosemary) marinated in Apple Cider Vinegar.

Fire cider gets its efficacy from the communal power of the sinus-clearing, warming, infection-fighting plants and a supplementary boost through the fermented **ACV**. This immune brew will burn (in a great way!) going down.

It is super easy to make, so make a batch and toss it on your salad every evening, sprinkle it on grain or quinoa, or take a shot when you can sense cold coming. If homemaking isn't your thing, you should find some from a local herbalist or at an all-natural food store.

Avoid using it if you have *Gerd*or a brief history of stomach ulcers.

6. Adaptogens

You've probably heard this wellness word buzzword in the last couple of years - adaptogens - but may not understand the exact thing it means.

"Basically, adaptogens are therapeutic herbs that assist the body to combat and adapt to stress. They're wonderful to use for those who fall sick often,", "or in times of heavy stress, travel, or exposure to pathogens (rather than daily maintenance or prevention)."

Ashwagandha, reishi (both incite the infection-fighting lymphocytes, or white blood cells) and holy basil (stimulates the disease fighting capability and also fights viruses) are good options for supporting the immune system.

Buy <u>Reishi</u> as a powder and mix it into anything you are eating or drinking; it's safe to take small doses (like a scoop of powder or perhaps a squirt of tincture). *Ditto for ashwagandha*, although stay away from ashwagandha if you're taking thyroid hormones like Synthroid.

Holy basil can be converted into infusion and sweetened with honey (don't take it if you're pregnant, though, says Corbett). Research various other options, get one of these few and find out which ones do the job.

Why Plants are Crucial to Your Immune System Capability

Eating junk food weakens your disease-fighting capability, makes you vulnerable to illness and sets you up for several problems.

A study published in the Journal of Traditional Chinese Medical Sciences discovered that children who were reported to eat a diet plan full of prepared high-sugar foods with plenty of meat and few vegetables were more likely to have problems with repeated respiratory infections compared to those who ate healthier.

On the other hand, avoiding processed and fried foods, increasing your intake of fresh vegetables, fruit, herbs, spices, and plant-based protein sources like beans and nuts can strengthen your disease-fighting capability.

To start with, plants provide a lot of fiber that helps to feed the bacteria in your gut and regularly flush your GI tract of parasites seeking to gain dominance. And, considering that 70% of the diseases fighting capability is in the gut, a healthy microbiome is important to remaining healthy generally, explains Dr. Rawls.

People who eat plenty of dietary fiber also have their lungs functioning effectively compared to those who don't include them in their diets, according to a study of nearly 2,000 adults published in the history of the American Thoracic Society. But plants' immune-boosting powers go beyond fiber.

Vegetables, fruits, and herbs are rich sources of phytonutrients, natural plant chemicals that work to assist the immune system so it can better resist and fight germs. While no one can explain the exact way the phytonutrients in plants work, it's likely they support communication between different parts of the immune system.

"Immune cells need to communicate properly for your complete system to work optimally,". These cells serve as messengers, sending information backward and forwards that help your body to release the proper white blood cells and launch a defense against an attack or invader.

Like humans, plants also have to deal with attacks from potentially harmful viruses and bacteria. What is different, though, is how they've developed what I call <u>an all-natural intelligence to fight</u> them.

"Plants have internal chemicals that counter the microbes - they have an innate ability to look after themselves," he says. Your immune system was designed to look after the body, but plants' phytonutrients aid. "Whenever you ingest the natural intelligence of plants and herbs, it increases your body's natural intelligence."

You can simply do this by eating lots of different types of plants, but some foods and herbs are particularly good at targeting and supporting the human immune system.

Blueberries

These nice berries contain more antioxidants than all the type commonly consumed fruit, including a high level of *flavonoids*. An assessment of 14 tests by researchers in New Zealand discovered that eating flavonoids, either through food, juice, or supplements, reduced upper respiratory infections by 33% weighed against controls, and it also beats down sickness by 40%.

One kind of flavonoid specifically - ***quercetin***, with a high concentration in dark blue and red fruits - has been proven to have potent antiviral properties, even helping to stop the virus from replicating and reducing the viral load and lung inflammation.

Other foods rich in *quercetin* and other *flavonoids* include apples, onions, and green tea extract.

To get your fill, add berries to smoothies, yogurt parfaits, and desserts, snack on apples, add onions to salads and sandwiches and drink green tea extract.

Turmeric

This bright-yellow spice common in Indian cuisine has been useful for medicinal purposes for a long time.

Curcumin, one of its main compounds, gives it its color aside from its immune-boosting potential.

Research suggests curcumin helps to activate white blood cells and deregulate proinflammatory cytokines. Also, it can help to enhance an antibody response and show microbiome balancing activity.

Similar to ginger, eating turmeric-spiced foods is a great way to include the plant in your daily diet, but supplements will deliver the largest value for your money.

Cordyceps

While it is technically not an "herb," this fungus is popular in TCM for treating fatigue, sickness, and many more. It naturally grows around the back of a particular species of caterpillar that lives in the mountains of Tibet, and historically, it had been used for famous emperors and royalty. Recently, research shows that cordyceps help to boost immunity against flu.

"Cordyceps has elements of immunomodulation and resistance to any kind of stress,". More specifically, it works by stimulating natural killer (NK) cells and macrophage activity, and also by enhancing cellular immunity.

Much like the Chinese skullcap, you can take double portions of cordyceps if you want a supplementary immune boost beyond everyday support: Take 450 mg once a day, then progress to 900 mg daily as required.

Andrographis

Although not a plant you take in, this plant native to India continues to be used for many years for different purposes, including its ability to support a healthy immune system. "For viral illnesses, I'd rate Andrographis as one of the best plants available,". (I recommend taking 250 mg to 500 mg of Andrographis per day.)

Research shows that supplementing with Andrographis significantly helps to reduce symptoms of the normal cold. Patients taking Andrographis extract reported a break from nose secretions, tiredness, sore throat, and sleeplessness just after two days than those going for a placebo, according to findings in the journal Phytomedicine. After four days, the Andrographis group also reported a substantial reduction in all symptoms, including cough and headache.

Mushrooms

While alternative and Eastern medicine practitioners have relied on mushrooms to help them fight illness for many years, modern-day researchers needed to discover how key *fungi phytonutrients* – especially *beta-glucans* - work to aid the immune system.

Beta-glucans are complex polysaccharides or sugars that reside in the cell walls of mushrooms, and they appear to act on immune receptors and activate various immune cells, according to a paper in the Journal of Hematology and Oncology.

"Any kind of mushroom you find at the grocery store or a local food market will do the job,".
"But *shiitake, maitake, oyster, lion's mane, and turkey tail mushrooms have the best immune benefits.*"
Another powerful mushroom: **Reishi**; Preliminary studies suggest *reishi mushrooms* help to regulate the immune system by increasing the number of immune cells and the production of communication-enhancing cytokines,

according to a study review in Integrative Medicine: A Clinician's Journal.

You won't find Reishi in food markets, you will only get it in supplement form; aim for 350 mg daily.

Garlic

Long used for therapeutic functions, garlic is well known for its ability to help balance the good and bad microbes in the microbiome (the total of all microbes in your body). Recent research shows garlic also helps to improve the disease-fighting ability by stimulating sure immune cells and regulating the secretion of *cytokines* - natural chemicals made by immune cells that help the disease-fighting ability communicate and function.

In a study, placebo-controlled report published in Advances in Therapy, participants took the garlic supplement or a placebo for 12 weeks from November to February. Throughout that time, not more than a third of individuals in the garlic group got colds, while almost everyone in the placebo group did. The placebo-takers were also vulnerable to several colds during the three months, and their symptoms persisted longer (5 days versus 1.5 for the garlic group).

You can add garlic to your food; especially in its raw form (check it out in salads and salad dressings). But you'd have to eat three big cloves daily to get the most out of it, so supplementing with garlic is a wise bet.

Black and Green Tea Extract

Sipping a hot cup of tea is comforting when you're under the weather; however, it can perform other functions aside from keeping you warm.

A report in the journal Proceedings with the National Academy of Sciences discovered that drinking five cups of black tea every day seems to supercharge T cells (a kind of white blood cell that plays an integral role in immune response). After fourteen days of drinking the tea, the cells produced ten times more ***interferon***, a chemical that actively fights viruses and helps to stop them from replicating. If you like green tea that will also help.

Aside from **quercetin** (the beneficial flavonoid in blueberries), green tea extract also has ***theanine***, an amino acid that research shows may use other polyphenols to supply your immune system the boost it needs.

Making this food and herbs an integral part of your daily routine - not only during cold and flu season, but year-round - can go a long way in supporting a solid and healthy disease-fighting capability.

Don't forget to get enough sleep, regular physical exercise, stress management, and a standard nutritious diet to reduce your vulnerability to infections altogether!

Broccoli Sprouts

Sprouts from baby broccoli plants contain high degrees of a phytonutrient called sulforaphane, which you can also get from cauliflower, Brussels sprouts, and other cruciferous vegetables. Early research showed that eating the sprouts could increase inflammation-fighting enzymes in the upper respiratory system.

More recently, a report published in the journal PLuS One suggested that people who drank a regular shot containing sulforaphane-rich broccoli sprouts have a resistance to the flu virus. The researchers noted several changes to the subjects' immune cells after administering a live flu vaccine in their nostrils. Later, those that have been drinking the broccoli-sprout shakes showed lower levels of the flu virus in their sinus fluids compared to those who drank a control shake with alfalfa sprouts.

The sprouts blend well in green smoothies and shakes, besides they make a very tasty addition to salads.

Chinese Skullcap

This species of flowering plant in the mint family is a "heat-clearing" and phlegm-removing herb in Traditional Chinese Medicine (TCM), a historical practice for preventing and treating various diseases. Its reputation originates from its purported anti-inflammatory and antimicrobial effects.

For instance, in a study in the *Journal of Ethnopharmacology*, researchers suggest the Chinese skullcap helps to reduce the expression of pro-inflammatory cytokines that play an important role in our inflammatory response and resistance to pathogens. Other research shows Chinese skullcap as helping inhibit the growth of bacteria like Helicobacter pylori and coagulase-negative staphylococci, a staph bacteria that majorly affects the skin.

To get the immune-supporting benefits of the Chinese skullcap, I recommend taking 450 mg once a day. Or, if you're feeling slightly sick or you think your immune system is under more pressure than usual, increase the total amount to 450 mg twice a day.

Japanese Knotweed

This Japanese native is a rich way to get resveratrol, the chemical compound in wine that gives the adult beverage its healthy reputation. While resveratrol is most likely known for its antioxidant powers and heart health-promoting properties, also its antibacterial properties.

Japanese knotweed can help to inhibit the growth of "bad" bacteria in your gut microbiome, where almost all the components of the immune system are found while increasing the growth of "good" gut bacteria, he explains. I suggest taking 400 mg a few times daily, with regards to the degree of immune support you will need.

Ginger

This spicy plant does more than suppress nausea (an advantage it's popular for). Ginger contains almost twelve antiviral compounds, including some that appear to be particularly effective against a typical cold-causing virus, according to some paper in the International Journal of Drug Development & Research.

Extracts from both ginger plant and root were also found to be effective against two pathogenic staph strains, says a report in the Journal of Microbiology and Antimicrobials. Supplements supply the strongest dose. Nevertheless, you can also use ginger to spice stir-fry dishes, eat it pickled, or brew some ginger tea.

Important Steps to Make it Work

Most people believe that herbal treatments don't work, and that is often because they aren't using enough.

A glass of cold-fighting tea blend daily is not likely to help the immune system flush out any offending bacteria, especially once the symptoms of the infection begin to manifest.

If you want to get the most from a tea, you must steep it for a longer period and/or use more herbal material (read: two or three tea bags per cup, or put everything in a French press and allow it to brew for 30 or more minutes).

The same applies to *tinctures* – when your condition is acute, you have to be taking a full dropper (or whatever the guideline on the tincture bottle says) every few hours or so.

When in doubt about the dosage (and if a particular herb will work with your body), consult a trained clinical herbalist, holistic doctor, naturopath, or other trusted sources related to natural medicine.

And always consult your doctor or even a pharmacist if you're likely to mix plant medicine with prescription drugs.

Above all, listen to the body before, during, and after any seasonal illnesses. The best medicine for illness is prevention.

While healthy means different things for everyone, there are some healthy habits you can adopt to help you resist winter infections.

You understand the drill: sleep, fresh foods when possible, exercise and/or hanging out, and staying hydrated. And if the cold should creep in, you have a lot of plant buddies to help you.

"No herb is upgraded for a healthy lifestyle". "It can be beneficial; however, it won't fix you. The body has a vital intelligence that is equipped to send you messages on what it needs. Pay attention to it."

Chapter 6

Healthy Minerals and Vitamins

Sadly, too many people don't eat enough fresh fruits, vegetables, and other foodstuffs we need to keep ourselves healthy year-round. You simply can't eat an orange or grapefruit and expect one quick burst of vitamin C to prevent a cold. A healthy disease-fighting capability depends on a balanced mix of minerals and vitamins, including healthy sleeping habits and regular exercise.

With some exceptions, *it's better to get your minerals and vitamins from food instead of in pill form*. Below are a few tips that can help you get the necessary minerals and vitamins that your immune system will need to work effectively.

Vitamin A

Foods that are saturated in colorful compounds are called carotenoids - <u>carrots, sweet potatoes, pumpkin, cantaloupe, and squash</u> - are examples of them. Your body transforms these *carotenoids* into vitamin A, and they come with an antioxidant effect to strengthen the disease-fighting capability against infections.

Vitamin C

You probably know about the relationship between the immune system and Vitamin C already, but do you know you can get Vitamin C from other sources aside from citric fruits?

Leafy vegetables such as <u>spinach and kale, bell peppers, brussels sprouts, strawberries, and papaya</u> are also good sources. Vitamin C is present in a lot of foods that so many people might not need to consider supplements unless a doctor recommends it.

Vitamin D

As stated above, it is better to get most of your vitamins from food; however, Vitamin D can be an exception to that rule. You can increase your Vitamin D intake through foods like oily fish (<u>salmon, mackerel, tuna, and sardines</u>) and processed foods such as <u>milk, orange juice, and cereals</u>. Many people have difficulty absorbing vitamin D from food, if you have a vitamin D deficiency, speak to your doctor about supplements.

Vitamin E

Like vitamin C, vitamin E is a powerful antioxidant that helps the body fight off infection. Almonds, peanuts, hazelnuts, and sunflower seeds are saturated in vitamin E. So are spinach and broccoli if you like to improve your intake during meals rather than opting for snacks.

This important vitamin - a part of nearly 200 biochemical reactions within your body - is crucial to how your immune system operates. Food rich in vitamin B6 are bananas, chicken white meat, and cold-water fish such as tuna, cooked potatoes, and chickpeas.

Folate/Folic Acid

Folate *is the natural form, while* **folic acid** *is the synthetic form*; often added to foods due to its health advantages. To get extra folate, include more beans and peas in your diet frequently, as well as leafy vegetables. You can even get folic acid in processed foods (check the label) such as enriched bread, pasta, grain, and other completely whole-grain products.

Iron

Iron helps the body to transport oxygen to cells, and it is in different forms. The body can easily absorb "heme iron," which is made up of poultry foods such as chicken, turkey, and seafood.

Do not fret vegetarians; you can get other types of iron in beans, broccoli, and kale.

Selenium

Selenium seems to have a strong influence on the immune system, like the ability to slow down the body's overactive responses to certain aggressive types of cancer. You'll find it in garlic, broccoli, sardines, tuna, brazil nuts, and barley among other foods.

Zinc

You'll find zinc in oysters, crab, liver and chicken, baked beans (skip the type with added sugar), yogurt, and chickpeas. Zinc seems to help decelerate the immune response and control inflammation within the body.

Frozen is okay

Depending on your geographical area and what season it is, you can't always have high-quality fresh produce. Keep this in mind: Frozen is okay. Manufacturers freeze frozen fruits and vegetables at "peak" ripeness; this means they'll pack similar vitamins and minerals as their fresh counterparts. Just choose plain frozen foods instead of those that have added sugars or sodium.

As the entire world reacts and reels in response to the COVID-19 pandemic with no known treatments or vaccines yet available, it could be comforting to learn that we now have some diet plans you can switch to that can enhance your immune function.

Doctors know about the importance of proper nutrition in bolstering cellular health and, consequently, immune health.

Immune Boosters

Some foods can provide the immune system with the essential boost it requires, especially during the current infectious crisis.

Here are some of the foods you can consider in this infectious period to give your disease-fighting capability a fighting chance.

Poultry

Chicken soup could very well be the typical "sick" food. Its origin dates back to 7,000 to 10,000 years ago and is from the domestication of fowl, likely in either ancient India or Southeast Asia.

The combination of beneficial ingredients in the chicken soup helps to make it the best immune booster. For instance, researchers show that chicken soup can prevent the transportation of neutrophils to areas of infection or inflammations in people that have symptomatic upper respiratory system infections.

Cysteine, specifically, is a component of chicken that is known to stop the movement of white blood cells and reduce the mucus associated with colds.

No set of immune-boosting foods will be complete without mentioning poultry, i.e. chicken or turkey.

All poultry is saturated in vitamin B6, and 3 oz contains as much as 50% of the daily recommended dose. Vitamin B6 is essential for the formation of fresh and healthy red blood cells. Chicken soup also includes vitamins A and C, magnesium, phosphorus, and antioxidants, which are very important to immune function.

The protein in chicken and turkey also provides amino acids, which are used by the body to create antibodies to fight infection. Also, boiling poultry to make soup releases gelatin, chondroitin, and other nutrients that help your gut and immune system. Chondroitin, for instance, is a crucial element of mucin that affects gut permeability and intestinal immune mediation.

<u>Although canned chicken soup is okay, but try to make chicken soup from scratch for the most immune benefits.</u> Your ingredients won't ever have to be processed, and you can easily control the quantity of salt you use. <u>Fresh is better!</u>

Almonds

Almonds are rich in vitamin E, which including vitamin C is an integral player in keeping your immune system healthy. It is also a potent antioxidant that is vital for the proper functioning of the immune system. If your T-cells have been damaged through oxidative stress, they can't provide an adequate immune response against whatever pathogen is attacking your body. Vitamin E also plays a significant role in T-cell differentiation.

A half-cup of almonds will provide you with almost 100% of the daily recommended amount of vitamin E. A small number of almonds is a great snack anytime, and you can add them to your cooking, for extra texture and flavor.

Mushrooms

Mushrooms are saturated in selenium and B vitamins, including riboflavin and niacin. Each is ideal for your disease-fighting capability. *Selenium, for instance, is an antioxidant that helps to reduce oxidative stress; lessen inflammation, and enhance immunity.* And vitamin B6 is known to aid significant biochemical reactions within the immune system.

Another plus? Mushrooms are saturated in polysaccharides, which are sugar-like substances that boost immune function. The polysaccharides in mushrooms connect to macrophages, neutrophils, monocytes, and dendritic cells - all major team players of the immune system. Polysaccharides work to improve and/or activate the immune reactions of the cells and increase the production of reactive oxygen species and enhance *cytokine* and *chemokine* secretion.

Shiitake mushrooms, especially, are a good choice because they're rich in B vitamins, vitamin D, selenium, niacin, and seven out of eight essential proteins.

Chaga mushrooms are also a fantastic immune-boosting choice. They have the best concentrations of antioxidants and also contain a high amount of zinc, which can be very important to immune function.

Mushrooms are a savory, delicious addition to any meal. For example, you can sauté them with onions as a side dish to any meal; or add them to salad, or simply eat them straight with just a little dip.

Garlic

Garlic is a crucial ingredient in just about any cuisine around the world. It provides the sulfoxide alliin, but when smashed or chewed, alliin becomes allicin.

Because allicin is usually unstable, it converts to sulfur-containing compounds, which are believed to supply garlic with its medicinal properties. Garlic is known to improve the ability of the immune system by stimulating macrophages, lymphocytes, natural killer cells, dendritic cells, and eosinophils. It does this by *modulating cytokine secretion, immunoglobulin production, phagocytosis, and macrophage activation.*

Garlic is easy to include in almost any meal. Use it when preparing roasts, chicken, lamb, and fish. As well as add it to grain or mashed potatoes while boiling to add a delicious, flavorful, and healthy kick to meals.

Citrus Fruits

Citric fruits contain vitamin C, an important micronutrient. It plays a role in the improved health of the immune system by supporting cellular functions in both innate and adaptive disease fighting capability.

For instance, vitamin C supports the epithelial barrier function against pathogens. It also enhances differentiation and proliferation of the important disease fighting capability superstars: B- and T-cells.

Vitamin C can also increase the production of white blood cells - lymphocytes and phagocytes - that protect the body against infections. Furthermore, vitamin C supplements can prevent and treat respiratory and systemic infections. Vitamin C also acts as an antioxidant, helping to fight free radicals that damage the disease-fighting capability and affects its proper functioning.

Vitamin C, however, isn't the only player in citrus fruits. Flavonoids - plant compounds that have anti-inflammatory, antioxidant, and free-radical scavenging properties and are other ingredients of citrus fruits that give the immune system a boost by helping to reduce inflammation and enhance speed recovery from sickness.

Because the body can neither produce nor store vitamin C, you must eat rich sources of vitamin C daily-especially if you are ill and your levels are depleted. <u>Citric fruits like</u>

oranges, tangerines, lemons, limes, grapefruits, and clementines are great sources of Vitamin C.

Other ways of adding some natural vitamin C to your diet include topping a salad with a squeeze of lemon or lime or adding a squeeze of any citrus fruit to a cup of plain water or even tea. All are easy ways to get your daily vitamin C fix.

But, if you're not a fan of citrus fruits-or detest some of the medications that could adversely connect to citrus fruits or citrus juice, consider taking vitamin C supplements, which are many and easy to find.

Pomegranates

The energy of pomegranates in immune health is multifactorial and has many "genres" of pathogens. Consider that compounds in pomegranate extract have been proven to inhibit the growth of parasites such as *Escherichia coli O157:H7, Salmonella, Yersinia, Shigella, Listeria, Clostridium, and Staphylococcus aureus.* Pomegranate extracts have also been shown to have antiviral properties that are effective against flu and other viruses. As if this weren't enough, pomegranate extracts are also used to promote the growth of beneficial gut flora- such as Bifidobacterium and Lactobacillus that can also give a powerful boost to your immune system.

Get the pomegranate ready by drinking as juice. You can even eat pomegranates completely, or sprinkle its seeds on salads or yogurt for a delicious change of diet.

Everyone understands that lemons, and other citric fruits, are rich in vitamin C, among many other nutrients. Recently, researchers all over the world have studied the effects of vitamin C as well as an essential and multi-functional role in human health. One area where it is known to play a major role is in the immune system.

Lemons and Zinc

A report by researchers in Switzerland in 2006 and published in the history of Nourishment & Metabolism examined both the role of Vitamin C and zinc in boosting the immune system, and whether that effect could apply to patients with specific conditions, such as respiratory tract infections, and the common cold, among others.

It is known that the level of vitamin C in the blood serum drops when the body is under physical or mental stress, or when under attack as a result of contamination. This is mostly because the body's immune system uses more Vitamin C when under attack by infection.

- Vitamin C improves the ability of natural killer cells, that help to get rid of infection, and assist in antimicrobial activity;
- It can help the body's supporting cells such as lymphocytes;
- It can help the body's cells maintain their strength, and resist oxidative damage.

Zinc also acts on specific components of the body's immune response; hence the two were studied together. Both nutrients are necessary for maintaining a healthy body.

- They help your body resist infectious diseases;
- They decrease the severity of the bout of infection;
- They decrease the amount of infection.
- Keeping you healthy.

The study examined the results of what it called a "lot" of tests where patients received up to 1g of vitamin C or more to 30mg of zinc. What they found was significant.

- Consumption of vitamin C and zinc improved symptoms;
- It had also been connected with a reduced period in the infection, disease, or condition.

This response was connected with several conditions, including:

- Respiratory infections;
- The normal cold;
- Pneumonia;
- Malaria;
- Diarrhea infections in children.

What does this mean?

Eating lemons - that have about 60mcg of zinc per 100g - and other citric fruits, helps to increase your disease-fighting capability and keep you healthy, and a supplementary boost can help if you are fighting a cold or other infection.

Orange Probiotic Immunity Boosting Smoothies

These Orange Probiotic immune-boosting smoothies are ideal for breakfast on the run. A vegetable and fruit-based yogurt smoothie rich in vitamin C, Vitamin A, fiber, and Calcium.

The other main component to make a probiotic smoothie, is, of course, the *probiotic-rich kefir yogurt*.

Kefir yogurt from either grass-fed organic dairy or non-dairy (vegan friendly). This vegan kefir yogurt is my fresh favorite. But allow me to deviate a while.

You will observe that kefir yogurt is produced from kefir "grains" by itself. These do not necessarily grain all the bacteria and yeasts that match the milk (dairy or non-dairy) to make a lightly fermented drink or yogurt drink, something like *kvass and kombucha*.

It can be made anyway to get milk, such as goat, sheep, cow, rice, cashew, or coconut. It can even be made with coconut water.

These *kefir* grains have a beneficial symbiotic combination of lactic acid bacteria and yeasts in a polysaccharide-protein matrix. I understand, super nerdy and science.

But to explain it briefly, this bacteria protein blend is packed with vitamins, nutrients, and can aid in increasing bone relative density, boost immunity, and improve digestion.

Studies have finally shown that even people who are lactose intolerant are made for kefir.

Ingredients for Smoothie

Okay, so back to the smoothie ingredients. The kefir yogurt, and super-foods below, lead to one ***Power Probiotic Rich Smoothie*** recipe. Let's go deeper into the other ingredients, shall we?

Fresh Orange - Vitamin C!!

Carrots - Well-known Vitamin A rich vegetable. And do you know Vitamin A is needed for supporting the line of the digestive system? Yep, you want to keep that gut lining working strong! It serves as an obstructive barrier for food-borne pathogens and the others in the body.

Dates - Abundant with potassium and Fibre.

Chia seed - Abundant with omega 3's, plant protein, and fiber.

Ginger and cinnamon- Suitable for digestion and super-foods.

Coconut oil (optional) - but can help you to absorb fat-soluble vitamins.

Kefir Yogurt - as explained above.

Healthy notes to remember => As much as I love to get probiotics from real food, we can't always get as much as we need. Such as, if I fall sick and need to consider an antibiotic, then my gut flora would become depleted because I have been wiping out all the bacteria, actually here is the good! Eating more probiotic foods and going for a probiotic supplement can help to rebuild that gut flora more efficiently. Both can work together to rebuild that gut flora.

Orange Probiotic immunity boosting smoothies are ideal for breakfast on the run. A vegetable and fruit-based yogurt smoothie rich in vitamin C, Vitamin A, fiber, and Calcium. No sugars needed.

Ingredients:
- One large carrot, peeled
- 2 tangerines or 1 large orange (regular or blood orange)
- 6-ounce of fresh orange juice
- 1 tsp chia seed (more if you're making smoothie bowls).
- 6-8 ounces simple Kefir yogurt or cultured natural yogurt.
- Three to four 4 dates, pitted
- 1/2 tsp Cinnamon
- 1/2 tbsp grated ginger
- 1/2 tsp vanilla (optional)
- Optional 1/2 tbsp coconut oil
- 2 cups (2 small bowls, or 1 large bowl).

Instructions:

- Peel your carrot and oranges.
- Place carrots, orange, and juice in a blender. Blend under a thick juice if formed.
- Next add your chia seeds, yogurt, spices, ginger, and coconut oil.
- Blend again.
- To create smoothie bowls, add an extra tsp of chia seed, and allow blended smoothie mix to cool for a while, (or at least for a couple of hours) in the refrigerator. The chia seeds can help it to thicken. Pour into bowls and garnish with orange slices, cinnamon, gluten-free oats, and optional honey.

Notes

This bowl of smoothie can serve as breakfast. Two small servings or one large. Adjust the sweetness to your desired taste, with the addition of optional honey or maple syrup. Mix into smoothies before serving.

For a vegan option, use coconut milk yogurt or Forager cashew kefir yogurt.

Smoothie Tips for Cancer Patients

When you have cancer, eating ideally can provide you with the strength you need. Smoothies are one of the ways to get the required nutrients the body needs to fight the condition and handle the side effects of treatment.

Smoothies are a good option in case your treatment has some side effects. Smoothies will also be cold, which can soothe a sore mouth and throat. If you're too tired to eat, or you don't have an appetite, drinking your calories can be a very perfect alternative.

Everyone has different nutritional needs; your doctor can help you identify yours. Knowing them, you should use these guidelines to prepare a nutritious and delicious smoothie.

Focus on Fruit

Fruit provides sweetness and fiber -- that aid your digestive health -- and disease-fighting antioxidants. Try mixing different fruits for several mixtures of nutrients and flavors.

If you have soreness in the mouth, try to avoid fruits with small seeds, like <u>berries</u>. The seeds could worsen your mouth injury.

You should use fresh or frozen fruit. If you need a thicker texture, choose frozen.

There are many good fruit options. Bananas are saturated in potassium; a mineral the body needs for the nerves and muscles to work effectively. Pears have lots of fiber, which can ease constipation. Mangoes contain vitamins A and C that make your disease-fighting capability stronger. Watermelon helps to hydrate you, and it also offers lycopene, a robust antioxidant. Cherries and other dark-colored fruits have chemical substances called phytochemicals that help to fight cancer.

Remember that cancer treatment could make your smoothies taste too sweet. If that's the situation, make an effort to include frozen cranberries, which add tartness.

Include Veggies.

Vegetables are a great way to obtain nutrients and fiber. They're also low in sugar which will help to keep your blood sugar levels in balance. Consider adding: Leafy greens, which provide B vitamins and iron. The body uses these to create blood cells. *Spinach, kale, and romaine lettuce are good options.*

Carrot and pumpkin are naturally sweet fruits that are saturated in vitamin A.

Avocado, which is also a fruit, is saturated in heart-healthy fats. It is also a good way to gain calories.

Then add Protein.

The body uses it to correct tissue and make your immune system stronger. Most times, people who have cancer need more protein than those who don't. It can help to heal tissue and fight off infection after and during treatments like surgery and chemotherapy.

Good resources of protein are:
- Nut butter or whole nuts.

- Unsweetened Greek yogurt.
- Protein powder.

Look for low-sugar protein powders, with things such as whey, hemp, rice, or peanut. A budget-friendly option is dry skim milk powder. Don't consume excess protein; the body can't process more than 30 grams of it at a time.

Pour in a few Liquids.

Smoothies can help you stay hydrated which is particularly important when you have nausea or diarrhea. Filtered water adds liquid without calories; besides, it creates a milder-tasting smoothie. Coconut water contains sodium and potassium so it replaces electrolytes. Low-fat milk is a good option if you wish to add creaminess and calcium to your smoothie. Plant-based milk, like almond, soy, oat, and rice milk are also alternatives you can consider.

Go for unsweetened options and the ones fortified with vitamin D and calcium. The juice is a superb choice if you wish to gain more calories. Look for varieties with 100% juice.

Give it Improvement.

Consider adding seeds, spices, or herbs to your smoothie for extra flavor and nutrition.

Ginger or mint can soothe stomach upset: Cinnamon, turmeric, and cardamom have anti-inflammatory compounds. Flax meal is saturated in fiber. Also, it contains healthy omega-3 fats. Chia seeds contain protein, fiber, calcium, and omega-3 fats.

Avoid the added sugars: It's a myth that sugar causes cancer to grow faster but added sugar provides extra calories without much nutrition. Mix the table sugar, honey, maple syrup, and agave. Fruit gives your natural smoothie sweetness.

Practice food safety: Cancer and certain treatments can weaken your immune system. This makes it harder to fight off disease-causing bacteria in contaminated foods. That is why you must handle and prepare foods carefully.

Ensure you:

- Wash your hands carefully.
- Make use of a cutting board reserved for fruits & vegetables.
- Ensure juices and milk are pasteurized.
- Scrub all raw vegetables & fruits with a brush and water before you cut, peel, or eat them. Especially those with hard peels like oranges and avocados.
- Soak fresh berries and frozen fruits & vegetables in water.
- Put any leftover smoothie in the fridge immediately.

Try these Mixes.

1 cup of filtered water

½ frozen bananas

½ ripe pears

½ Granny Smith apples

2.5 cups spinach

Juice of ¼ lemons

2 cups of frozen unsweetened blueberries

½ cup of calcium-fortified orange juice

¾ cup of low-fat or non-fat vanilla yogurt

½ medium frozen bananas

½ teaspoon of pure vanilla extract

1 mango, peeled and cut into chunks

½ orange, peeled and quartered

1 carrot, sliced into chunks

1½ cups of unsweetened soy milk

1-inch little bit of ginger, peeled

6 ice cubes

1 cup of unsweetened vanilla almond milk

½ cup of brewed green tea extract

1½ tablespoons of ground flax or chia seeds

½ teaspoon of fresh minced ginger

¼ teaspoon of cinnamon

1 tablespoon of lemon juice

½ cup of berries

½ cup of banana or mango

2 cups of spinach or kale

1 tablespoon of almond butter.

Chapter 7

Immune-Boosting Recipes

Runny noses, aches, chills, and severe coughs fits are probably not one of ways you intend to spend your fall. Yet, there you are, under the covers and cold to the bone. Not hungry. No energy. Wondering what you are going to do while you're before you are fit to go out again.

You can cook anything. Even though no food sounds appealing to you but food can actually be a magical thing. It can work to nourish you and increase your disease-fighting capability meaning you will have to spend fewer days on your sickbed. While sick, you will be wishing that your nose will clear so you can breathe again and have the opportunity to spend time outdoors enjoying the gusty fall air.

There are at least fifteen well-balanced meals on our diet plan to improve your immunity. These recipes contain most of them. Ensure you try out some of these meals and you will realize your immune system will get the nutrients it requires to defend the body against potential illness and cure anyone that is currently affecting the body.

California Salmon

Ingredients:
- 3 cloves garlic, minced
- 1 teaspoon minced shallot
- 1 cup of orange juice
- 1 tablespoon balsamic vinegar
- 3 tablespoons honey
- 1 tablespoon ground ancho chile pepper
- 1/4 teaspoon salt
- 1/8 teaspoon pepper
- one 16-ounce salmon fillet
- 2 teaspoons canola oil
- 2 tablespoons minced cilantro

Instructions:
- In a little saucepan coated with cooking spray, sauté the garlic and shallot until tender. Add the orange juice and vinegar and allow it to boil. Reduce heat; simmer, uncovered, for 20-25 minutes or until

reduced to ¼ cup. Add the honey, chile pepper, salt, and pepper.
- Preheat the oven to 400 degrees.
- In a big ovenproof skillet, brown salmon in the canola oil on both sides. Brush with ¼ cup from the sauce. Bake uncovered for 8-10 minutes or before the fish flakes easily with a fork. Brush with remaining sauce and sprinkle with cilantro.

Chicken Noodle Soup

There is nothing that can be compared with chicken noodle soup, and sometimes circumstances warrant a big, large plate of it. Put in a little brown rice or quinoa to make this into a meal, or simply serve it as has warm crusty bread.

Ready in 32minutes

8 Servings, 526 Calories Per Portion

Ingredients:

- 2 salted butter
- 1 large onion, sliced finely
- 1/2 salt
- Two 32-ounce cartons of low-sodium chicken broth

- 1 pasta, such as ditalini
- 10 frozen mixed vegetables, such as peas, carrots, corn, and green beans
- One 15-ounce can of diced tomatoes
- 6 cooked boneless skinless chicken breasts, chopped
- 1 grated Parmesan
- 2 lemon juice
- 1/4 black pepper
- 1/4 chopped chives (optional)

Instructions:

- Melt the butter in a big stockpot over medium-low heat. Add the onion and ½ teaspoon in the salt. Cook, stirring often, before the onion is soft and translucent, for about ten minutes.
- Bring the broth and allow it to boil over high temperature. Stir in the pasta, frozen vegetables, and tomatoes. Cook before the pasta is ready, for about 7 minutes.
- Stir in the chicken, Parmesan, lemon juice, remaining salt, pepper, and chives. Cook for a

minute more to heat through, remove from heat, and serve.

Superfood Salad

Yield: 1 serving Prep time: 5 minutes, Total time: 5 minutes.

A superfood salad with ginger, garlic, parsley, and lemon to keep you healthy and fit throughout the year.

Ingredients:

- Half an inch of ginger
- 1 small garlic clove
- Small couple of parsley
- 1 carrot
- 1 small beetroot
- 1 kale leaf
- 1 small celery stalk
- 1/2 lemon
- 1/2 ripe avocado
- one to two 2 teaspoons hemp oil
- 1/2 teaspoon toasted sesame oil
- Sprinkle of sea salt

- Sprinkle of hemp seeds.

Instructions:
- Finely grate the ginger (without skin).
- Crush garlic (remove skin).
- Finely chop parsley.
- Grate carrot and beetroot.
- Chop kale leaf.
- Chop celery.
- Juice lemon.
- Cube avocado.
- Put hemp seed oil and sesame oil.
- Sprinkle salt.
- Mix everything and top with hulled hemp seeds.

Enjoy!

Citrus Glazed Roasted Carrots

Lemon and orange juices add a bright citrus **note to** roasted carrots. The honey glaze brings out the natural sweetness in carrots. This recipe comes from the Delight of Kosher.

Ingredients:
- 2 pounds carrots, peeled

- 2-3 tablespoons essential olive oil
- Kosher or sea salt
- Fresh cracked black pepper
- 2 large lemons, 1 halved and 1 juiced
- 2 small oranges, 1 halved and 1 juiced
- 4 tablespoons honey
- 1 teaspoon dried thyme.

Instructions:

- Preheat the oven to 425 degrees F.
- Peel and slice the carrots in a straight manner into fours or sixes, based on the size of the carrots.
- On a big, lightly greased sheet pan, toss the carrots with the essential olive oil, salt, and pepper. Place the halved lemon and cut orange side up in the pan as well, and roast until tender for about 20 to 25 minutes. Keep a careful watch as the cooking time will vary based on the size of the carrots.
- Remove from the oven and toss with honey, thyme, and the rest of the orange and lemon juice.
- Go back to the oven and cook until caramelized and lightly charred for about 10 minutes to quarter-hour. Serve warm or at room temperature with the roasted citrus halves.

Broccoli Rabe and Kale Harvest Salad

Ingredients:

Broccoli Rabe and Kale Harvest Salad

- 3/4 cups farro, rinsed
- 2 cups of water
- 1 couple of broccoli rabe
- 1 couple of lacinato/dino kale; about 5 packed cups of chopped kale
- 1 small fennel bulb
- 1 small sweet apple, such as a gala or honey crisp
- 1 small red onion, roughly ¼ cup of thin slices
- 1/4 cup ¼ cup walnut halves, toasted and chopped
- Orange-Cranberry Dressing
- scant 1/2 cup frozen whole cranberries, thawed
- 1/4 cup extra essential olive oil
- 1/4 cup fresh orange juice
- 1 tablespoon orange zest
- 1 inch of fresh ginger, peeled
- 1 tablespoon pure maple syrup
- Salt and pepper, to taste

Directions:

Broccoli Rabe and Kale Harvest Salad

- In a medium saucepan over medium heat, mix the rinsed farro, 2 cups of water, and a pinch of salt. Allow the farro to boil for a while, cover the pot and reduce the heat to a simmer.
- Cook the farro for 20 minutes, or until it's cooked but still has a little that can be chewed. Drain the farro and keep.
- Rinse out the saucepan which you used for the farro and fill it with about 2 liters of water. Place the pot over medium heat. Allow it to boil slightly. Set up an ice bath in a mid-sized bowl.
- Trim the tough stems from the broccoli rabe and cut them into bite-size pieces. Drop half of the cut broccoli rabe into the saucepan and place the lid on it right away. Allow the rabe to steam for approximately 3-4 minutes, or until tender and lightly wilted.
- Transfer the steamed broccoli rabe into the ice bath. Continue this blanching procedure with the rest of the broccoli rabe.

- Remove this because of the kale and chop the leaves into bite-sized pieces. Place the chopped kale into a large bowl. Scrape the fennel bulb, reserving a number of the fronds, and take away the core. Scrape the fennel with a mandolin on the bowl using the kale. Remove the apple core and trim it with a mandolin in the large bowl. Remove the tough outer peel with the red onion and scrape it with a mandolin above the large bowl.
- Squeeze all the excess water from the blanched broccoli rabe and stick it in the large bowl with the kale along with other shaved fruits/vegetables. And add the cooked farro to the bowl.

Orange-Cranberry Dressing

- To make the dressing, mix the thawed cranberries, essential olive oil, orange juice, orange zest, fresh ginger, maple syrup, salt, and pepper in a straight blender. Blend the mixture on high until you might have a smooth consistency.

- Season the salad with salt and pepper and pour 3/4 of the Orange-Cranberry dressing into the salad.

Massage the dressing into the kale, broccoli rabe, farro, and other fruits & vegetables until everything is equally coated. Transfer the dressed salad into a big platter. Drizzle the rest of the dressing at the top and garnish the salad with the cut walnuts and fennel fronds.

Tuscan Broccoli-Tomato Tarts

Ingredients:

- 1 refrigerated pie crust, such as Pillsbury™, softened as directed on box
- 1 egg white, slightly beaten
- 11-ounce bag frozen broccoli, such as Green Giant™ Steamers™ Tuscan seasoned broccoli
- ½ cup shredded sharp Cheddar cheese (about 2 ounces)
- ¼ cup mayonnaise
- ¼ cup chopped red onion
- ⅓ cup chopped sun-dried tomatoes in oil, drained in writing towels.

Instructions:

- Preheat the oven to 400 degrees F. Unroll a pie crust on the work surface. Use a 2-inch round cutter, cut 24 rounds through the crust, rerolling the dough as necessary. Press 1 round underneath or more the sides of every 24 ungreased mini muffin cups; brush lightly with the egg white. Bake for 8 minutes.
- Meanwhile, microwave the broccoli as directed by the package; drain. Cool slightly, and then chop finely. In a little bowl, mix the cheese and mayonnaise.
- Spoon slightly less than ½ teaspoon on the onion and about ¼ teaspoon from the tomatoes into each cup. Top with 1 tablespoon broccoli (cups will be full). Spoon about 1 teaspoon of the mayonnaise mixture together in each cup.
- Bake before the crust is light golden brown and the cheese melts, for about 16 to 20 minutes. Immediately remove from the pan to a serving plate. Serve warm.

Applewood Smoked Salmon with Warm Potato-Apple Salad and Ale Dressing

You should be eating salmon throughout the year, but it's especially important during flu season. The omega-3 essential fatty acids increase the activity of macrophages, the white blood cells that destroy bacteria in your body.

Ingredients:
- 1½ pound red potatoes, cut into 3/4-inch chunks
- 4 tablespoons essential olive oil
- 2 Golden Delicious apples, cored and cut into 3/4-inch chunks
- 4 frozen salmon fillets, such as Sea Cuisine Applewood Smoked Salmon
- ½ cup pale ale or lager beer
- 5 tablespoons cider vinegar
- 1½ teaspoon salt
- 1 teaspoon sugar
- 4 scallions, sliced
- 1 tablespoon Dijon mustard
- ¼ cup chopped fresh parsley

Instructions:

- Preheat the oven to 350 degrees F. Mound the potatoes on the rimmed baking sheet. Drizzle it with 1 tablespoon of the essential olive oil; toss to coat and spread evenly around the sheet. Bake for 20 minutes. Scatter the apples around the potatoes and bake until tender, for a quarter-hour or more.
- Meanwhile, cook the salmon based on the package instructions.
- Mix the ale, 3 tablespoons of vinegar, salt, and sugar in a big skillet. Set over medium heat and allow to a boil. Add the scallions and simmer for three minutes.
- Remove from heat and whisk in the mustard. Whisk in the rest of the 3 tablespoons essential olive oil and 2 tablespoons vinegar until blended.
- Add the potato mixture and parsley to the skillet; toss to coat. Serve with the salmon.

Gingered Carrot-Orange Soup

Ginger aids in stimulating pancreatic enzymes that help you to stabilize your blood sugar levels and burn food as fuel, not storing it as fat.

Ingredients:
- 4 cups organic vegetable broth
- ½ cup coconut aminos
- 2 cups chopped carrots
- 1½ cup sliced red onions
- 1½ teaspoon ginger paste
- 2 15-ounce cans of garbanzo beans, drained and rinsed
- 3 oranges, peeled and halved
- Peel of ¼ orange
- ⅛ teaspoon ground cinnamon
- Pinch of ground nutmeg
- Pinch of ground coriander
- Sea salt and black pepper to taste
- 6 slices sprouted-grain bread, toasted
- 6 cups fruit.

Instructions:

- Heat a non-stick skillet over medium heat. Put ½ cup from the broth along with the coconut aminos in the skillet and heat slightly. Add the carrots, onions, and ginger paste and cook, stirring, for approximately ten minutes or before carrots and onions are soft.
- Transfer to some mixing bowl. Add the rest of the broth, beans, oranges, orange peel, cinnamon, nutmeg, coriander, and salt and pepper.
- Pour into a blender in batches until smooth. Transfer the soup to a big pot and heat gently. Serve the soup hot, it has a slice of toast and 1 cup of fruit per portion.

Grilled Salmon with Mediterranean Salsa

The salsa can be prepared ahead - store it in a tightly sealed container and refrigerate for a long time or overnight. Put in a simple grilled salmon that must only be cooked for ten minutes, and you'll understand why the efficiency of the recipe has a spot in our assortment of Best Salmon Recipes.

Ingredients:

- 1/2 cup cut fresh parsley
- 1/3 cup sliced plum tomatoes
- 1/4 cup ATHENOS Traditional Crumbled Feta Cheese
- 1/4 cup coarsely chopped pitted kalamata olives
- 2 tablespoons essential olive oil
- 1 tablespoon lemon juice
- 4 salmon fillets (4 ounces each)

Instructions :

- Preheat grill to medium heat. Mix parsley, tomatoes, cheese, olives, oil, and lemon juice until well blended. Allow it to stay at room temperature until ready to use.
- Grill salmon for five minutes on each side or until salmon flakes easily with a fork.
- Serve each fillet topped with 1/4 cup in the tomato salsa.

Healthy Potato, Spinach, & Pumpkin Seed Hash

Filled with heart-healthy foods like spinach, pumpkin seeds, and mushrooms, this *"hypertension awareness hash"* is ideal for a balanced and healthy diet. Besides, it is also delicious!

Ingredients:

- 3 cups small new potatoes, cut into two
- Olive oil
- 1/4 teaspoon freshly ground black pepper
- 1/4 teaspoon smoked paprika
- 1/4 cup unsalted pumpkin seeds
- 1/4 teaspoon whole black peppercorns
- 4 cloves garlic, roughly chopped
- 3 loosely packed cups spinach
- one 15-ounce can no-salt-added chickpeas, rinsed
- 1/4 teaspoon dried dill
- 2 cups mushrooms, like cremini, oyster, or perhaps a mixed variety.

Instructions:

- Preheat oven to 375 degrees.
- Place the potatoes over a rimmed baking sheet. Drizzle 2 teaspoons of olive oil on the potatoes, add the pepper and paprika and ensure the entire pan is covered and shimmy before the potatoes are covered up with oil and spices.
- Place the potatoes in the oven and cook until brown and soft for about 30-35 minutes.
- Warm 2 teaspoons of essential olive oil in a skillet over medium heat. When hot, add the pumpkin seeds and toast for 5-8 minutes. Add the black peppercorns and the garlic and cook for another five minutes.
- Put the pumpkin seeds, peppercorns, and garlic into a food processor. Add the spinach and 1 tablespoon of olive oil, and pound until all the ingredients form a creamy pesto. Put in a few glugs (a supplementary tablespoon roughly) of essential olive oil as needed. Put your pesto aside.

- Once the potatoes are cooked, place them in a bowl, and cover with foil to retain the warmth. Then increase the heat of the oven to 425 degrees.
- Put your garbanzo beans around the baking sheet in one layer and place them into the oven to roast for ten minutes. Remove the beans from the oven, add the dried dill, shake the pan, and cook for 8-10 minutes.
- As the beans cook, reheat your skillet, and add another teaspoon of essential olive oil when the pan is dry, so when hot, add your mushrooms so that they are in a layer. Let them cook uninterrupted until brown for about 5-8 minutes. Then stir and let them cook for another 5-8 minutes.
- To serve, gently mix the crispy garbanzo beans and the mushrooms with the potatoes. Then, spread the pesto on each plate and layer the potato, mushroom, and crispy garbanzo hash at the top. Dig in and enjoy!

Blueberry Orange and Almond Pancakes With Orange Maple Glaze

Breakfast during intercourse, anyone? It gets even cozier with the nourishing antioxidants and vitamin C-filled glaze.

Ingredients:

For the pancakes

- 1 all-purpose flour
- 1 granulated sugar
- 1 baking powder
- 1/2 baking soda
- 1/2 salt
- 1 large egg
- 3/4 buttermilk
- 1/4 fresh orange juice
- Scant 1/4 teaspoon almond extract
- 1/2 to 3/4 cup fresh blueberries (or frozen, thawed, and drained)
- 3-4 butter, for griddle or pan

For the glaze

- 1/2 powdered sugar

- 3 fresh orange juices
- 1 pure maple syrup

Instructions:

For the pancakes

- Place a rack in the third upper part of the oven and preheat the oven to 200 degrees. The oven will keep the pancakes warm while you bake them in batches.
- Inside a medium bowl, whisk flour, sugar, baking powder, baking soda, and salt together. In a little bowl, whisk egg, buttermilk, orange juice, zest, and almond extract together.
- Whisk the buttermilk mixture into the flour mixture until it is well mixed. Put in the blueberries. Let batter rest for five minutes as the griddle heats.
- Over medium heat, melt 1 tablespoon in the butter in a cast-iron skillet or griddle. Spoon 2 tablespoons batter into the hot pan and cook until golden brown on both sides, about 2 minutes per side.
- Place pancakes with an ovenproof dish and store them in the oven to remain warm while you cook other batters, adding butter to the pan as needed.

For the glaze

Whisk powdered sugar, orange juice, and maple syrup together. Serve alongside warm pancakes. Pancakes are best served immediately.

Indian-Spiced Tomato and Black Bean Soup

For a good way to add spice to traditional tomato soup, add warm Indian spices and black beans.

Ingredients:

- 2 tablespoons of grape seed oil
- 1 onion, chopped
- 4 garlic cloves, minced
- 1 teaspoon of grated ginger
- 2 serrano chiles, seeded and diced
- 1 teaspoon of coriander
- 1 teaspoon of cumin
- 1 teaspoon of paprika
- 1/4 teaspoon of turmeric
- 1/4 teaspoon of cinnamon
- 28 ounces of plum tomatoes, peeled
- 4 cups cooked of black beans
- 2 teaspoons of salt

- 1 teaspoon of black pepper
- Sour cream, for garnish
- Cilantro leaves, for garnish.

Instructions:

- In a big pot, heat the oil over medium-high heat. Sauté the onions until translucent for about five minutes. Add the garlic, ginger, and chiles, and cook for 2 minutes. Add the coriander, cumin, paprika, turmeric, and cinnamon. Cook for another 2 minutes.
- Stir in the tomatoes along with the black beans. Bring to a boil, reduce heat, cover, and cook for approximately 10 minutes. Using a spoon, break apart the tomatoes until they are in large chunks. Season with salt and pepper. Cook for another 10 minutes for flavors to meld.
- Garnish with a dollop of sour cream and cilantro leaves.

Foil-Baked Cod with Oranges, Scallions, and Ginger

An instant and satisfying recipe for supper. The citrus with this recipe complements the fish perfectly! It is an instant and easy option for a delicious evening (or weekend) meal.

Ingredients:

- four 6-ounce cod fillets
- 1 cup sliced scallions
- 2 tablespoons coconut aminos (or low-sodium soy sauce)
- 2 tablespoons toasted sesame oil
- 1 tablespoon finely minced fresh ginger
- Zest and juice of just one 1 orange
- 4 oranges, peeled and sliced
- Salt and pepper.

Instructions:

- Preheat oven to 450 degrees F. Tear off 4 large sheets of foil.
- Place one cod fillet on each of the foil sheets.
- Season fish with salt and pepper.
- In a medium bowl, mix the scallions, coconut aminos, sesame oil, ginger, and the zest and juice of just one 1 orange.

- Pour together with the cod fillets, distributing the dressing consistently between the four bits of fish.
- Top each fillet with 3-4 orange slices.
- Fold the ends of the foil together tightly, ensuring that the packets are completely sealed.
- Place them on the baking sheet.
- Bake the cod for 12-14 minutes, or before fish is opaque and easily flakes apart.
- Take away the packets in the oven, and let them cool for approximately 5 minutes.
- Season with additional salt and pepper to taste.

Serve and enjoy!

Jerk Shrimp and Citrus Salad

The dish was made to bring a few of my roots (Jamaican pepper shrimp) into a more sophisticated healthy meal. Pepper shrimp in Jamaica is street food sold in little bags on the road, so with just a little flair and some dose of my type of consuming (light and salad-type foods), the homey favorite became an extremely refreshing and healthy meal ideal to be served on a hot day.

2 Servings, 609 Calories Per Portion

Ingredients:

- 1 tablespoon balsamic vinegar
- 1/4 cup plus 2 tablespoons essential olive oil
- 1 grapefruit, segmented, juice reserved
- 1 orange, juice reserved
- Salt and freshly ground black pepper, to taste
- 1/2 pound shrimp, peeled and deveined
- 1 tablespoon hot jerk seasoning
- 1 small red onion, julienned
- 1/2 pound beets, roasted and cut into wedges
- 6 ounces cucumber, peeled and sliced
- 2 heads baby lettuce, preferably organic.

Instructions:

- In a bowl, mix the balsamic vinegar, essential olive oil, and 1 ounce of juice from the grapefruit and orange. Season with salt and pepper to taste. Whisk to make the dressing and keep.
- In another bowl, marinate the shrimp in the jerk seasoning for a quarter-hour. Meanwhile, preheat a grill over medium heat. Then, toss the shrimp with 2 tablespoons in the dressing and grill for 2 minutes on each side.

- Add the red onion, beets, cucumber, and baby lettuce to a bowl and toss with the rest of the dressing. Place the salads in 2 equal portions in 2 bowls, and add the citrus segments and shrimp. Season with pepper to taste.

Tomatillos

Ready in 1 hour

4 Servings, 296 calories per portion

Ingredients:

Chop

- 3 pounds Tomatillos
- 1 Green Bell Pepper
- 4 tablespoons of olive oil
- 1 pinch of salt
- 3 ounces of Blanco Tequila
- 1 White or Yellow Onion
- Cook
- Blender

Instructions

- Chop

- Remove the skin and the stems of the tomatillos, and then slice into two.
- Cut onions and bell pepper with a food processor.
- Cook
- Saute tomatillos in essential olive oil until soft.
- Blend all of the ingredients in a food processor until smooth.

Chicken with Garlic and Parsley

This recipe makes chicken succulent and simple. A profile of rustic Italian flavors, both refined and simple, takes this classic dish from the chef's kitchen to yours.

4 Servings, 222 Calories Per Portion

Ingredients

- 12 cloves garlic, peeled
- 1/4 cup Italian parsley leaves
- Salt and freshly ground black pepper, to taste
- 4 chicken white meat halves, boneless, skin-on
- 2 tablespoons unsalted butter
- 1 large lemon, juiced
- 1 tablespoon parsley, finely chopped

Instructions:

- In a little saucepan, blanch the garlic cloves in boiling water for 1 minute. Drain water and cut the garlic thinly. In a little bowl, toss the garlic with the parsley and just a little salt and pepper.
- Stuff a small amount of this garlic mixture into the pockets under the skin with the chicken breasts (about 2 teaspoons per chicken). Transfer the chicken to a plate, cover with plastic wrap and chill until it is ready to be used.
- Heat a charcoal or gas grill until it is moderately hot. Grill, the chicken for 8 to ten minutes per side before the meat is cooked thoroughly. Do not overcook it. Once you're done, remove the chicken from the grill.
- Over medium heat, melt the butter in a sauté pan and gently sauté the rest of the garlic mixture. Add the lemon juice and chopped parsley and season to taste with salt and pepper.
- Pour this sauce into the plated, cooked chicken.

Roasted Garlic Kale Hummus

If you're looking for a creative way to use super-nutritious kale, try making a hummus-style dip from it. It has beautiful bright green color and is packed with garlic and tahini flavor.

Ingredients:

- 7 cloves garlic, roasted
- 15-ounce can garbanzo beans, drained
- 1 cup tightly packed kale leaves
- ¼ cup fresh lemon juice (about 2 lemons worth)
- 2-3 tablespoons water
- ¼ cup tahini paste
- ½ teaspoon salt, or even to taste
- Essential olive oil, for serving.

Instructions:

- Preheat the oven to 400 degrees F. Wrap the garlic cloves (with the skin on) in aluminum foil and place inside the oven to roast for 20 minutes. Allow the garlic to cool before peeling off the skin.
- Put all ingredients into a food processor and blend until smooth.

- Serve the hummus with essential olive oil drizzled at the top and with pita bread or more fresh vegetables.

Roasted Sardines, Lemongrass, and Tomatoes

Ripe tomatoes and fresh lemongrass bring new heights of flavor to these baked sardines. Serve on toast for a straightforward and elegant appetizer! A white wine from Côtes de Bordeaux is best to play with the flavors with the fish.

Notes

- Wine Pairings
- Traditional pairing: Pair with a fruity and mellow Bordeaux dry white from Côtes de Bordeaux.
- Non-traditional paring: Choose on a fruity and mellow Bordeaux nice white from Côtes de Bordeaux.

Ingredients:

- 3 stalks of fresh lemongrass
- 2 very ripe tomatoes cut into small pieces
- 4 cloves garlic, minced

- Olive oil
- Thyme
- 18 sardines gutted and scaled
- 6 slices white bread.

Instructions:
- Place the sardines in a baking dish (only 1 layer).
- Bake at 400 degrees F for ten minutes, turning over after five minutes.
- Add the tomatoes, lemon-grass (cut in two lengthwise), garlic, thyme, and salt and pepper. Pour into an oiled pan.
- Simmer quarter-hour over medium heat.
- Around the slices of toasted bread, place a layer of tomatoes after removing the stalks of lemongrass.
- Top with a layer of sardines.

Rosemary Citrus-Herb Turkey

Ingredients:

- 1/3 cup thinly sliced garlic cloves
- 1/3 cup fresh rosemary
- 2 tablespoons fresh thyme
- 2 tablespoons mild essential olive oil
- 1 teaspoon salt
- 1 teaspoon cracked black pepper
- Grated peel of just one 1 lemon
- Grated peel of just one 1 orange
- 10- to 12-pound turkey, such as JENNIE-O, thawed, giblets, and neck removed

Instructions:

In a food processor, add the garlic, rosemary, thyme, essential olive oil, salt, pepper, lemon zest, and orange zest together; process this before removing the peel of the citrus and garlic and also before the ingredients are well blended. Refrigerate until prepared to use. Rub the herb mixture on the surface of the turkey. Roast turkey according to package directions.

Spaghetti Squash and Zucchini

Some people only think about sautéeing these vegetables with a little butter, but this recipe demonstrates how far both can go when cooked with fresh basil, Parmesan cheese, and toasted pine nuts. Perfect as a salad or like a side dish for your holiday meal.

4 Servings, 215 Calories per servings.

Ingredients:

- 1 cup spaghetti squash
- 1 cup julienned zucchini, with skin on
- 1/2 cup broccoli florets, blanched
- 1/2 cup julienned roasted red pepper
- 1 teaspoon chiffonade basil
- 1/4 cup extra-virgin essential olive oil
- 1/4 cup water
- 1 teaspoon lovely butter
- 1 teaspoon each salt and white pepper
- 1 tablespoon toasted pine nuts
- 1 tablespoon shredded Parmesan cheese
- 1/2 cup plum tomato sauce
- 1 tablespoon extra-virgin essential olive oil, to drizzle by the end of the dish

Instructions:

Heat a sauté pan to medium heat and add water and essential olive oil to bring to some simmer. Bring the red peppers and zucchini to cook for 2 minutes. Add spaghetti squash, broccoli, and cauliflower. Season with salt and pepper and cook for two minutes. Add the butter until melted, after then add basil.

In the second sauté pan, heat the plum sauce to a simmer. The sauce can be held warm. Spoon the tomato sauce into a pasta bowl, making a large circle in the middle of the plate. Mound the spaghetti squash mixture, in the middle of the plate. Sprinkle with Parmesan cheese and pine nuts. Drizzle oil over the top and around the dish and serve.

Spinach Orange Smoothie Recipe

Here is a thick, creamy, and healthy smoothie recipe.

Natural greens are capable of supercharging your entire day like nothing else. Spinach, kale, and arugula smoothies help alkalize the body, while simultaneously providing energy-boosting antioxidant support.

Blend a small number of leafy greens and watch the magic happen.

Ingredients

- 1 navel orange, peeled
- 1/2 banana
- 1 cup tightly packed organic spinach
- 1/4 cup coconut water, adjusted as desired
- 1 tablespoon hemp seeds, optional
- Ice.

- **Instructions:**

  Add all ingredients into a blender with a few pieces of ice and blend on high to mix. Add more coconut water according to your desired consistency for a smoothie.
- Pour into a glass and enjoy!

Middle Eastern Spiced Cauliflower Soup

Get cauliflower when you feel under the weather – it is rich in glutathione, a potent antioxidant that helps to fight off infection, and besides, supports a solid disease fighting capability with *vitamin C and selenium*. This spicy soup will ensure your health is in the best condition especially during winter, with a lot of spices and a dollop of yogurt.

Stir-fried fish with chili, ginger, and eggplants

Antiviral and antibacterial, the medicinal properties of ginger have been exploited for many years. Like a diaphoretic, it encourages perspiration, increases your intake if you're having symptoms of fever like cold and flu. This fragrant dish is packed with tasty vegetables to keep you fit.

Braised Beef with Fire-Roasted Green Chilies

A small amount of beef in your diet can go a long way, this nutrient-rich food contains protein for muscle growth, zinc to help to create a healthy disease-fighting capability, and iron to aid in transporting oxygen within the blood. Strengthen your health through winter with this simple and hearty dish.

Spinach gratin

Popeye may have placed it in the spotlight but the medical benefits of spinach are worth the fuss. Saturated in iron, which plays a major role in the operation of red blood cells that help to transport oxygen around the body, spinach is a good way to obtain *vitamin K, folic acid, magnesium, and vitamin B2*. Make this simple gratin for lunch or as a satisfying side dish.

Crisp Eggplant with sweet-spiced yogurt and Pomegranate

Probiotics, the live, active cultures in yogurt, help to keep the guts free of disease-causing germs.

Some studies have discovered that yogurt might be effective in boosting immunity, and it is more delicious compared to daily probiotic pill!

This sweet and spicy dish is loaded with all the benefits that can provide a healthy bacteria boost.

Soy, Ginger, Cumquat, and Gin Oysters

Shellfish such as oysters, crabs, lobsters, and clams contain selenium, which aids white blood cells to produce cytokines - proteins that help to rid the body of the flu virus. These tasty little bites also contain ginger, garlic, and chili and they are packed with immunity-boosting goodness.

Slow-Cooked lamb Kashmir Shanks

Warm and peppery, turmeric is mostly known because of its bright yellow color as a staple in most curries. Used for several years as a potent anti-inflammatory in Chinese and Indian medicine, this super-spice is an all-natural antibacterial. Try out this tasty recipe for a nutritious boost, its spice mix is filled with health-enhancing ingredients.

Porridge with Spiced Poached Apple

Oats contain beta-glucan, a kind of fiber with antimicrobial and antioxidant capabilities stronger than echinacea. Also, they are filled with *avenanthramides*, which perform strong antioxidant activities and increase our immune system's reaction to bacterial infection. Make this porridge your go-to meal on a cold morning and something to keep you full and warm at night.

Stewed Green Beans with Tomato, Chili, and Cinnamon

Rich in antioxidants, *cinnamon is known to suppress the growth of bacteria and contain anti-inflammatory properties.* This easy Italian dish is a tasty way to include a small amount of this powerful spice in your daily diet, but experience might make you sprinkle some on your oats, coffee, pumpkin soup… every tiny bit counts!

Thai-Style Lemongrass and Chili San Choy Bau

Just like its flavor, a small amount of chili can go a long way in helping to maintain your health. Traditionally found in Mayan medicine, hot peppers have always been valued for its antimicrobial and antibacterial qualities, and one recent study in China discovered that regular consumption of spicy foods had an inverse relationship with certain factors causing death. Although, as the authors described, it had been an observational report, and more research will be needed to draw inferences. However, there is something to be said for eating something which has a kick if you are feeling a little down with cold and flu symptoms! These spicy dishes are fast and simple to make, and also a very important thing if you sense weakness.

Celeriac, Potato, and Roast Garlic Soup

Garlic is essential in each winter grocery list - not only does this pungent veggie adds a big flavor boost; it also provides a lot of health-enhancing benefits. While there is still a lack of strong evidence about the effect of garlic on colds, we do know it contains antioxidants such as *vitamin C and quercetin*, and also the important compound *allicin*. Enjoy this thick, creamy soup during winter and enjoy all the benefits of this kitchen staple. Celeriac, potato, and roast garlic soup.

Meyer Lemon, Butter Mushroom, Fennel and Radicchio Salad with Parmesan

Citrus fruits such as lemons, limes, and oranges are filled with vitamin C, which is important for a healthy immune system. Research suggests Vitamin C can help to prevent cold for those under physical stress. Lemons are versatile; however, we particularly love the freshness they bring to the salad.

Vegetarian Pho with Shitake Mushrooms

There is much to love about mushrooms, aside from the fact that they are powerful immunity boosters. A University of Florida study showed increased immunity in individuals who ate a cooked shiitake mushroom every day for one month. This tasty broth also has cinnamon, ginger, and chili and is an ideal meal when you slightly feel under the weather.

Stuffed Sweet Potatoes

With regards to protecting your body from parasites, our skin is the first barrier and it needs vitamin A to keep it healthy.

One of the ways to ensure you're getting enough Vitamin A is to eat a diet plan rich in **beta-carotene**.

One of the best resources of *beta-carotene* is the humble sweet potato. This easy dish can also be served as breakfast.

Chicken and Spelled Soup

Chicken soup is wonderful for more than just the soul. Tests by the University of Nebraska Infirmary discovered that chicken soup can ease the symptoms of upper respiratory system infections. If you sense a cold coming, snuggle up with this classic comfort dish.

Conclusion

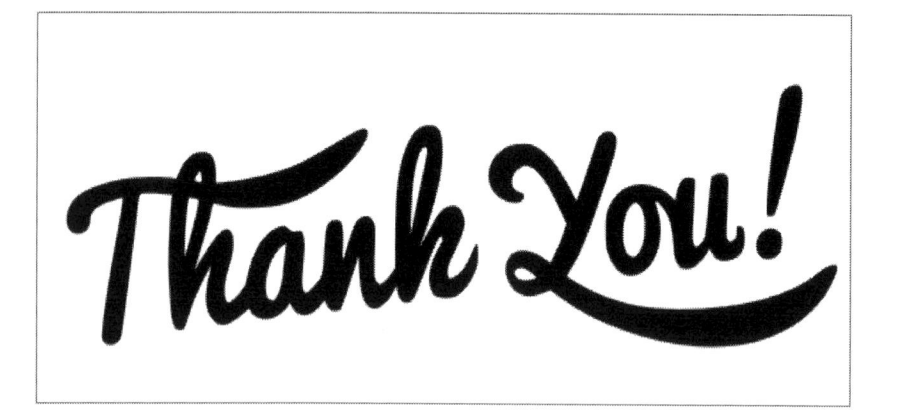

I'd like to express my gratitude for reading this book, **Thank You** for purchasing this book. I hope this book was helpful to you?

Your feedback as to whether I succeeded or not is greatly appreciated, as I went to great lengths to make it as helpful as possible.

I would be grateful if you could write me a review on the product retail page about how this book has helped you. *Your review means a lot to me, as I would love to hear about your successes.* Nothing makes me happier than knowing that my work has aided someone in achieving their goals and progressing in life; which would likewise motivate me to improve and serve you better, and also encourage other readers to get influenced positively by my work. Your feedback means so much to me, and I will never take it for granted.

[Click here to write me a review on how this book has helped you!](#)

or visit the product retail page to post your success story.

However, if your feedback is negative, it is possible that you are not impressed enough, or you have a suggestion, errors, recommendation, or criticism for us to improve on; we are profoundly sorry for your experience (remember, we are human, we are not perfect, and we are constantly striving to improve).

Rather than leaving your negative or displeasure feedback on the retail product page of this book, please send your feedback, suggestion, or complaint via E-mail to **"feedback@read.engolee.com"** so that action can be taken quickly to ensure necessary correction, improvement, and implementation for better reader experience.

I want you to enjoy your reading experience; your satisfaction is my number one (#1) priority. We will promptly make amends, and get back to you.

Thank you once again for reading this book, have a wonderful day!

Recommended Books

Below you'll find some of my other popular books on Amazon, including other authors books. Simply click on the links below to check them out.

If the links do not work, for whatever reason, you can search for these titles on the Amazon website to find them.

Dr. Sebi Alkaline Diet: The Complete 30-Day Meal Prep Cookbook with Over 100 Alkaline Based Food Delicious Recipes

Cabbage Soup Diet Recipes: The Quick Weight Loss Program's Guide For Men and Women

Anti-inflammatory Diet: The Cookbook for Preventing and Reversing Inflammatory Symptoms and Diseases Naturally, to Promote Healthy Living (Healthy Eating Lifestyle Movement)

Dash Diet Mediterranean Cookbook: 150 Food Recipes and Solution for Boosting Metabolism, Weight Loss, and Blood Pressure

The Complete Plant Based Diet Cookbook: with Over 80 Everyday High Protein Delicious, and Healthy Whole Food Recipes (Healthy Eating Lifestyle Movement)

Weight Loss Guide: The Cabbage Soup Diet Cookbook

Atkins Diet Cookbook: The Life Changing Diet Plan to Shed

Excess Weight by Eating Right, and Not Less; Suitable for Beginners and Dummies

Dr. Sebi: Alkaline Diet Cookbook For Beginners: The 30 Day Meal Plan Plant Based Diet and Meal Prep Guide: Dr. Sebi Recipes Book

Meditterean Diet Cookbook: The Cabbage Solution Diet For Easy and Quick Weight Loss

Anti-inflammatory Diet for Beginners: The Complete Solution for Healing and Boosting Immune System with Healthy Foods, and Recipes for Longevity

The Anti-inflammatory Diet Meal Prep : The Complete 101 Meal Plan and Recipes for Healing the Immune System (Autoimmune Issues and Inflammation) for Beginners

Over 150 Dash Diet Recipes for Dummies and Beginners: The Blood Pressure (Hypertension and Hypotension), Weight loss Solution Action Plan Cookbook

The Complete Plant Based Diet Cookbook for Beginners: 100 Delicious, Healthy Whole Food Recipes To Cook Quick & Easy Meals

Dash Diet For Beginners: The Complete Diet Plan Cookbook for Weight Loss, and Blood Pressure with Balanced Foods for Healthy Living

The Plant Based High Protein Diet Cookbook: The 101 Delicious Everyday Recipes for Beginners

Cabbage Soup Diet Recipes: The Quick Weight Loss Program's Guide For Men and Women

The Complete Plant Based Diet Cookbook: with Over 80 Everyday High Protein Delicious, and Healthy Whole Food Recipes (Healthy Eating Lifestyle Movement)

BONUS: (Free Books)

Books are the best and most efficient way to learn something new, it is our life-blood. Through the power of books, we connect with each other, evolve as a society, and find our purpose.

Join the community of over a million and growing enthusiasts readers committed to the literary life, and be among the first to receive notification when I and several Authors have special deals, giveaway, and also ARC (Advanced Readers Copy) of our book(s), and you'd be pleased to sign up to the **Exclusive List** to get access to your **FREE BONUS BOOKS**.

Here are a few of the Free books you'll get:
- CBD For Beginners.
- Overcome Imposter Syndrome.
- Power Of Visualization.
- Superior Brain Health.

…and many more!

To get instant access to these Free books, and community that will send ARCs, and book deals to you, click the link below:

Click here to **Download** Your **FREE BOOKS**.

Or visit the URL https://read.engolee.com

It's an amazing, and growing community where they share helpful tips and resources to help in your journey towards healthy living, wealthy lifestyle, getting entertained with good fiction stories, and more.

Printed in Great Britain
by Amazon